# Praise for *Outside the Womb*

*Rae and Riley offer a thorough, thoughtful look at the complexities of assisted reproduction from philosophical, theological, and scientific points of view. This book provides answers to the mind-boggling questions raised by new developments in reproductive technology. It's a resource I recommend highly.*
>    CHUCK COLSON
>    The Colson Center for Christian Worldview

*A rare blend of scientific information, biblical guidance, and empathy for those struggling with infertility. You won't find a better or more readable resource.*
>    DAVID STEVENS, MD
>    Chief Executive Officer, Christian Medical and
>    Dental Associations

*In addition to the emotional anguish experienced by couples with infertility, the treatment options now available through assisted reproduction present them with both a moral and scientific minefield. Scott Rae and Joy Riley do a superb job of unraveling the mystery and navigating the reader through this minefield.*
>    GENE RUDD, MD (obstetrician/gynecologist)
>    Senior Vice President, Christian Medical Association

*If you are looking for moral guidance on assisted reproduction that combines empathy with ethics, biblical teaching with contemporary application, and simple explanations with profound insights regarding IVF, IUI, GIFT, ZIFT, egg donation, surrogate motherhood, and prenatal genetic testing, then you've come to the right place. Congratulations to Drs. Rae and Riley for an outstanding contribution!"*
>    JOHN F. KILNER, PhD
>    Professor of Bioethics and Contemporary Culture and
>    Director of Bioethics Programs, Trinity International
>    University

*Where Catholic thinking has long been present in a theological ethic of the body, Rae and Riley make much-needed contributions that greatly add to the debate from a Protestant point of view. While their views on assisted reproductive technologies differ from my own,* Outside the Womb *is a thought-provoking and timely encouragement to think carefully and critically about these matters.*

JENNIFER LAHL
President, the Center for Bioethics and Culture Network

# Outside
## the
# Womb

| Moral Guidance for
Assisted Reproduction |

Scott B. Rae & D. Joy Riley

**MOODY PUBLISHERS**
CHICAGO

All Scripture quotations, unless otherwise indicated, are taken from the *Holy Bible, New
International Version*®, NIV®. Copyright ©1973, 1978, 1984 by Biblica, Inc.™ Used by
permission of Zondervan. All rights reserved worldwide.

Scripture quotations marked NASB are taken from the *New American Standard Bible*®,
Copyright © 1960, 1962, 1963, 1968, 1971, 1972, 1973, 1975, 1977, 1995 by The
Lockman Foundation. Used by permission. (www.Lockman.org)

All websites listed herein are accurate at the time of publication but may change in
the future or cease to exist. The listing of website references and resources does not
imply publisher endorsement of the site's entire contents. Groups and organizations
are listed for informational purposes, and listing does not imply publisher endorsement of their activities.

Information in the text does not in any way equate to medical or legal counsel.

Edited by Pamela J. Pugh
Interior Design: Smartt Guys Design
Cover Design: DogEared Design
Cover Image: iStock

**Library of Congress Cataloging-in-Publication Data**

Rae, Scott B.
 Outside the womb : moral guidance for assisted reproduction / Scott B. Rae, D. Joy
Riley.
   p. cm.
Includes bibliographical references.
 ISBN 978-0-8024-5042-5
 1. Human reproductive technology—Moral and ethical aspects. 2. Human repro-
ductive technology—Religious aspects—Christianity. I. Riley, D. Joy. II. Title.
RG133.5.R34 2010
618.1'7806--dc22
                    2010028641

We hope you enjoy this book from Moody Publishers. Our goal is to provide high-
quality, thought-provoking books and products that connect truth to your real needs
and challenges. For more information on other books and products written and
produced from a biblical perspective, go to www.moodypublishers.com or write to:

Moody Publishers
820 N. LaSalle Boulevard
Chicago, IL 60610

1 3 5 7 9 10 8 6 4 2
*Printed in the United States of America*

# Contents

**PART I: Laying the Foundation**

1. The Experience of Infertility. . . . . . . . . . . . . . . . . . . . . . . . . . . . . . . . . .11

    Definitions of terms . . . . . . . . . . . . . . . . . . . . . . . . . . . . . . . . . . . . . . .23

    Overview of the book . . . . . . . . . . . . . . . . . . . . . . . . . . . . . . . . . . . . . .33

2. Theology of Family and Procreation. . . . . . . . . . . . . . . . . . . . . . . . .37

3. Catholic Natural Law and Procreation . . . . . . . . . . . . . . . . . . . . . .55

4. The Moral Status of Fetuses and Embryos. . . . . . . . . . . . . . . . . . .77

**PART II: Evaluating Procedures**

5. Intrauterine Insemination and Egg Donation . . . . . . . . . . . . . . . 107

6. GIFT, ZIFT, and IVF . . . . . . . . . . . . . . . . . . . . . . . . . . . . . . . . . . . . . . 131

7. Surrogate Motherhood . . . . . . . . . . . . . . . . . . . . . . . . . . . . . . . . . . . . 163

8. Prenatal Genetic Testing . . . . . . . . . . . . . . . . . . . . . . . . . . . . . . . . . . 197

Afterword. . . . . . . . . . . . . . . . . . . . . . . . . . . . . . . . . . . . . . . . . . . . . . . . . . . 225

Notes. . . . . . . . . . . . . . . . . . . . . . . . . . . . . . . . . . . . . . . . . . . . . . . . . . . . . . . 229

Acknowledgments . . . . . . . . . . . . . . . . . . . . . . . . . . . . . . . . . . . . . . . . . . . 245

# PART I:

# Laying
## the
# Foundation

The Experience of Infertility

Theology of Family
and Procreation

Catholic Natural Law
and Procreation

The Moral Status of
Fetuses and Embryos

*Undoubtedly, infertility is one of the most*

*painful things a person and a couple can experience.*

# CHAPTER ONE

# The Experience of Infertility

The faces of infertility are many and varied. Sometimes the most surprising one is seen in your own mirror. At first, getting pregnant is just something you're waiting to have happen. After all, a couple doesn't always become pregnant with the first several attempts. A few weeks pass. Then it is a niggling little reminder at the back of your thoughts. Could this be a problem? Months pass.

Friends are having children, and conversations in which you once felt included now only isolate you. For some reason, you cannot bring yourself to *ooh* and *aah* over the latest positive pregnancy test, labor and delivery story, or nursing or diapering ecstasy. Holidays when families gather have become difficult, and Mother's and Father's Day are actually painful.

By the time one year of having unprotected sexual intercourse without pregnancy passes, a couple has met the criteria for infertility.

Infertility statistics are just that—statistics—until those numbers include the person in the mirror. In addition to the difficulties of the holidays with family members and their children and the ever-shrinking list of friends in similar circumstances, there are problems in unexpected places.

## Jake and Mandy

Jake and Mandy Anderson's story is a case in point. In their early thirties, they had been trying for a year and a half to have a baby, without success. They had seen their doctors. Mandy's tubes were clear of blockage and Jake's sperm count was satisfactory. Mandy was checking her temperature for a rise denoting ovulation. She called Jake whenever that happened. More than once, he had had to interrupt his workday for what initially seemed a romantic rendezvous. Over time, the pleasurable and gratifying sex life they had anticipated became something they never imagined. It seemed at times a chore, and was always a reminder of the fact that they were unable to conceive. Mandy would typically be in tears when her period began each month. They even wondered out loud if having a child was worth going through all of this, and contemplated a life without children. Together, they started looking into adoption as an alternative, but found they were still not quite ready to give up trying to have a child of their own.

Another unanticipated experience, which made their infertility even more difficult, was the way it affected each of their self-images. For Mandy, so much of being a fulfilled woman was bound up with having a child. Not that she would lose her identity in her child's, but she had a deep longing to conceive and experience childbirth and the bonding with her newborn that her friends talked about with such intimacy. She felt somehow less of a woman because she was failing to achieve one of her most significant callings in life.

Jake felt his manhood and virility were threatened; what kind of man was he if he couldn't impregnate his wife? Whatever they had expected, it certainly was not this level of soul-searching brought on by the clinical-sounding word—infertility.

After two years of frustration, Jake and Mandy reached a turning point. They consulted an infertility specialist one of their friends recommended. It was not without fear and trepidation. They had heard about the expense of fertility treatment. They had also heard some cautionary advice from Marc, their pastor. He seemed concerned that infertile couples were not trusting God to give them a child, but Mandy and Jake were confident that they had trusted God through the process so far, and they had prayed consistently as they tried to get pregnant. Marc thought that many infertility treatments were "unnatural." This bothered Jake and Mandy, too, but then, taking one's temperature in order to know when to have intercourse was a bit odd. Marc was hesitant about using any procedure that would involve another person to help a couple conceive and bear a child. These thoughts and more were in the backs of the Andersons' minds as they consulted Dr. Walters.

Dr. Walters was empathetic with their situation. He expressed more care for them than had many of their well-meaning Christian friends, whose advice had been basically to trust God or accept childlessness as His calling for them. The infertility specialist explained that there were a variety of reproductive technologies available, with the only constraining factor being their ability to pay.

He told them about a dizzying alphabet soup of techniques. There was IUI, DI, GIFT, ZIFT, IVF, and ICSI to name a few. Some were very expensive, and they did not know how they could pay for them. But others involved less money, so that was encouraging.

The doctor explained that some of these techniques would involve genetic materials from only the two of them. But others included a third person contributing either genetic material (the egg or the sperm) or the womb in which the child would be gestated. In some cases, a woman might even provide both egg and womb.

They left the meeting with the doctor, encouraged that their situation was far from hopeless, but also very confused about which treatment or treatments to try.

## Another Couple

Jake and Mandy are only one of several fictitious, but typical couples you will meet in this book. No couple represents any real persons, but Jake and Mandy could have been named Scott and Sally Rae. We struggled with infertility for several years. Although we did eventually conceive and bear three children, our journey through infertility touched

---

### TECHNOLOGY AND INFERTILITY

In the past thirty years more than one million babies have been conceived by means of in vitro fertilization. While assisted reproductive technologies are advancing, there is an ongoing battle to overcome the problem of maternal age and infertility. One technology that offers a ray of hope for combating the problems of maternal age is known as vitrification. Vitrification allows doctors to flash-freeze unfertilized eggs so that the woman can postpone pregnancy to a later age. A study in Spain revealed that the rates of success with in vitro fertilization do not differ between using a frozen and a fresh egg. This procedure is helpful for young women who want to preserve eggs for later in life, but there is not much that can be done for women who have diminished fertility, generally women past the age of thirty-five. However, frozen eggs are more sensitive to temperature and hence less reliable than frozen embryos and sperm, and as a consequence vitrification is not a widely used process; doctors generally only recommend this procedure for cancer patients who undergo treatments that will leave them sterile. In the end of the day, assisted reproductive technologies may be progressing, but scientists can't do much to alter the fact that women's fertility diminishes with age.

Source: Leslie Berger, "Racing to Beat the Maternal Clock," *The New York Times*, Dec. 12, 2007, NYTimes.com.

us deeply and changed us in ways we could not have imagined.

We have had other struggles as well. Recently, I asked Sally to compare the pain of infertility to what she experienced in her successful battle with breast cancer (radical surgery, reconstruction, chemotherapy, and so on). She replied *without any hesitation* that the pain of infertility was much more difficult to endure. She and I both remember vividly the pain we experienced, and believe that we can offer genuine empathy and sound advice to infertile couples, as well as those who advise them.

### Bearing Advice

Long before a couple considers the technologies that are primarily the focus of this book, they talk to close friends, family members, or a professional, such as their pastor or a counselor. These confidants can offer a listening ear and a compassionate shoulder on which to cry, both of which are quite valuable. But frequently well-meaning individuals can actually increase the pain by the advice they give. Suggestions such as "just relax, you're trying too hard," or "it's just not the right time," often do more harm than good because they inadvertently communicate to the couple that their struggle is not that significant.

What may be worse are the spiritualized words of "encouragement" that tell a couple to trust in God, or that a couple may be childless because God has some other purpose for them. Both of the above may be true, but when offered as advice, it often seems callous and unfeeling, and a denial of the pain that the couple feels.

### Is This Book for You?

If you are a couple struggling with infertility, we've written this book for you to help you navigate the confusing world of reproductive technology. This book is also written for those who know a couple like Jake and Mandy, and want to help. If you are a professional or layperson who is involved with infertile couples and has at some time found yourself wondering, as a Christian, what to say to a couple contemplating some of these technologies, this book is for you.

Reproductive technologies often make headlines; not so, the ramifications of using them. Deeper consideration is needed. If you are teaching a class in your church, or in a college or graduate school on social issues, medical ethics, or reproductive ethics, then this book is for you and the people in your class. We have tried to make a very complicated subject understandable to people who may be thinking seriously about this for the first time, while at the same time helping the professional grapple with the complexity of the issues involved.

We have tried to analyze reproductive technologies from the perspective of a Christian worldview to help you draw some conclusions about which are morally allowed and consistent with biblical ethics. First are some basic issues that need to be addressed for the infertile couple.

## Spiritual and Emotional Aspects of Infertility

### Infertility Produces Real and Deep Pain

For couples who strongly desire a child, the inability to have one produces a strange mixture of emotions—anger, frustration, and disappointment, which may reach the point of despair after a prolonged struggle with infertility. Being around families, especially those with babies or young children, may make this more acute. The Christmas season can be particularly difficult for infertile couples, who may prefer to spend time by themselves or get away. Public or church celebrations of Mother's and Father's Day are painful reminders of desires unfulfilled.

One of the main reasons that infertility causes so much pain is that the ability to produce a child is at the heart of many people's gender identity. Whether it is a man's inability to father a child or a woman's inability to become pregnant, both men and women struggling with infertility feel like failures. The sense of inadequacy can be overwhelming at times. It can produce anger and resentment at the partner who is the "problem." To the infertile couple, we would say,

"Do not minimize the pain you are suffering. Resist those who would subtly encourage denial of the anguish you feel. Spend your time with those people who can empathize with you and encourage you."

For others, there are several platitudes as well as questions to be avoided. These include, but are not limited to, the following.

"Have you considered that God might not want you to have children?"

"If you adopt, then you'll get pregnant."

"All you need to do is relax; then you'll get pregnant. That's what happened to 'X.'"

"Whose fault is it?"

"What kind of undershorts do you wear?"

### It Helps to Share Your Thoughts and Feelings about Your Struggle

During this time, both of you will be bubbling cauldrons of emotion. It is not helpful to keep these emotions bottled up inside of you. Men frequently have a difficult time talking about infertility and sharing how they feel about it. The more you can encourage this kind of discussion, allowing for breaks from it from time to time, the better.

It is certainly appropriate and helpful to talk with another person of the same gender, and to get together with other couples who are in the same position as you. There are many support networks available for infertile couples, either through your church (you may even encourage your pastor to start one if your church does not have one already) or through a counselor or therapist in your community. RESOLVE is a national support network for infertile couples, and Christian groups such as Stepping Stones[1] and Focus on the Family can provide additional resources.

It is important to be honest with God with your feelings about infertility. Many couples are angry at God and doubt His sovereignty over them and His loving care for them. The psalmists in the Old Testament were extremely honest with God with their feelings, and there is never any indication that God thought any less of them for being so honest. To question God and to express anger at Him is not unusual for infertile couples who believe that God has a family in His plan for them. Many couples feel let down that God has not kept His promises to them. Many infertile couples would make wonderful parents, and it is not clear sometimes what God is doing in their lives.

## INFERTILITY SUPPORT SERVICES

There are groups available to many couples to provide support and encouragement in the journey of infertility. RESOLVE is the national infertility support network that provides information on all infertility treatments and advocates for public policy that supports these treatments. They also have local chapters around the country that serve as support networks for infertile couples. They support infertility awareness week in the spring of each year and provide resources for newer options such as embryo adoption. See their website at www.resolve.org for more resources they have available. A Christian version of RESOLVE, Stepping Stones, provides distinctly Christian-based support and information on infertility, helping couples stay in touch with their faith through the journey of infertility. They provide similar resources for support and information (www.bethany.org/step). A further resource is found on the American Society for Reproductive Medicine website (asrm.org).

## Resist the Urge to Focus on "Why?"

Whenever a couple or an individual experiences a trauma or difficult time in life, the natural and obvious question is "Why is this happening to me?" For a Christian, there is a bit of a twist to the question when they ask, "What is God trying to teach me through this time?"

For the infertile couple, as for anyone enduring hard times, this question may be unanswerable this side of eternity. Although some infertility may be the result of a sexually transmitted disease, often infertility does not fit into a category that readily answers the why question. Even if the root cause of a couple's infertility can be medically pinpointed, the medical cause does not normally answer the deeper question of "why?"

Though it is true that infertility—as well as all illnesses or difficulties—is a result of the entrance of sin into the world, it is not normally the case that infertility is the result of some specific sin of a particular couple. Ecclesiastes 3:11 helps put the why question into perspective. Solomon writes, "He has made everything beautiful in its time. He has also set eternity in the hearts of men; yet they cannot fathom what God has done from beginning to end."

Similarly in Ecclesiastes 11:5, with a figure of speech particularly appropriate for infertility, he writes, "As you do not know the path of the wind, or how the body is formed in a mother's womb, so you cannot understand the work of God, the Maker of all things."

These verses indicate that there are significant limits to what human beings this side of eternity can know about the plan of God for their lives, especially how things fit together into a coherent whole. It is much like viewing an Oriental rug, but from the underside. When we look at the rug in that way, we will see knots and loose ends and can only faintly make out the pattern. But when we see the rug from on top, we can see the intricate design in all its fullness and beauty.

Until Christ returns, we see life, and especially infertility, from the underside of the Oriental rug of God's plan. That view, and our inability to answer why will not change until we meet Christ face-to-face. Thus it is not a fruitful way to expend emotional energy, and it can be presumptuous to suggest such an answer to a struggling infertile couple. The more fruitful questions are "How can we cope with this?" and "Where can we get support in this?" rather than spending a good deal of emotional energy trying to unscrew the inscrutable and answer the unanswerable question: "Why?"

### Don't Let Desperation Cloud Your Judgment

There is little doubt that by the time many couples seriously consider some of the more expensive reproductive options, they have become desperate to have a child. Getting pregnant can become practically an obsession for them. To be sure, this springs out of a natural inclination to procreate, and the sense of desperation is understandable because of the way that infertility strikes at a person's sense of gender identity.

But it is also true that this desperation can lead couples to do things that they would not otherwise do. For example, it is not uncommon for people to go deeply into debt in a pursuit of the latest round of reproductive technology. It is also not uncommon for couples to be totally engrossed in this process, some to the point of not being able to take care of other important aspects of life. Though I would want to be very careful in talking to an infertile couple about this sense of desperation, it may be an appropriate concern.

The desperation to conceive a child needs to be evaluated in light of some important biblical virtues. Trust in God's care for and sovereignty over a couple is an important aspect of developing Christlike maturity. Patience, long-suffering, courage, and endurance are other significant Christian virtues that are sometimes compromised in the process of countering infertility.

This sense of desperation for a child and the feeling that a couple is not complete without one should not be taken as a given, but rather be brought to the light of Scripture. This is not to add further to the guilt and frustration that many infertile couples feel. Indeed, anyone who counsels an infertile couple and mentions their desperation should have earned the right to say things like these through their commitment to the couple and their consistent support of them in the process.

These are not questions to be brought up prior to the couple understanding your commitment to them and unconditional love for them. But support and love for a couple sometimes involves pointing out things about which they may not be aware. The virtue of the couple in the process of infertility does matter, and these questions should be faced, though never used as a club to bludgeon the couple into further guilt.

## COMING TO TERMS WITH INFERTILITY

In contrast to the technological message of society and the infertility industry to always keep going, some couples opt out of the infertility race and come to terms with their infertility. Pamela Tsigdinos, who with her husband tried various infertility treatments for roughly eleven years, wrote a book about the experience, entitled, *Silent Sorority: A (Barren) Woman Gets Busy, Angry, Lost and Found.* She has moved on without success at infertility treatments, and has accepted that additional attempts at procreating a child would bring potential for more heartbreak with a small chance at success. Diane Allen, director of the Toronto-based Infertility Network, said, "Many fertility clinics treat couples long after their financial and emotional bank accounts are overdrawn. It isn't often that I've heard of clinics trying to help patients gain acceptance that their fertility may be at an end."

Source: Adriana Barton, "When Couples Come to Terms with Infertility," *Vancouver Globe and Mail*, May 23, 2010, theglobeandmail.com.

### Set a Limit on How Far You'll Go

In light of the fact that couples normally become more desperate the further into the process they go, it is helpful to decide at the outset how far you will go. Moral parameters should help you set these boundaries, as well as financial and emotional considerations. To be sure, you should not make any final decisions until all the medical facts are ascertained.

Because of your strong desire for a child, you are in a vulnerable position when it comes to making decisions about how far to take the process. Many couples can be persuaded to give it one more try, when the chances may not be any better than on the previous tries. Certainly the one more try may produce a child, but statistically, the chances of conception after repeated failures are not high. But the frustration rate and the total expense increase with every try that does not result in a pregnancy. So while you are at the beginning of the process and therefore more objective, try to set some limits on how far you will go in pursuing different reproductive options.

One of the hardest decisions you may make in your life is the decision to stop employing assisted reproductive technology after you have been at it for some time, thus accepting childlessness or pursuing adoption as alternatives. But it may also be one of the wisest.

## *Walking Together*

Undoubtedly, as we have said, infertility is one of the most painful things a person and a couple can experience. Those who have not experienced it personally have a difficult time identifying with those who cannot conceive the child of their dreams. If you are currently infertile, our hearts go out to you. We hope the encouragement of this chapter and the general guidelines of this book are helpful to you.

If you are in the position of walking with friends of yours through infertility, we hope this helps direct you into ways that can be both helpful and encouraging to them. Please appreciate how intense is their struggle and how deep is their pain. Allow them to share their feelings with you without being judgmental of them, and especially without offering pious platitudes that will likely alienate you from them. Pray consistently for them, for ultimately it is God who opens the womb. In spite of all our sophisticated technology that enables us to peer into the womb, it is still the "secret place" over which God alone has ultimate control.

In the definitions and discussions that follow in this book, it should not be construed that medical advice is being given. I, Dr. Riley, am an internist by training, with a graduate degree in bioethics. I am not, nor have I ever been, an expert in infertility. My husband and I have experienced sorrow in miscarriages, and have walked with a number of friends through deeper waters of prolonged infertility. My hope in helping write this book is to make some of the terminology more understandable, and to help frame the discussion of the ethics involved in considering reproductive technologies.

## Definition of Terms

Louise Joy Brown, the world's first test-tube baby, was born on July 25, 1978. Research into reproductive technologies was suddenly in the public eye, and has since seeped into our consciousness, as further technological advances have been made. When used successfully, these technologies represent the miracle of life for couples who have often spent years trying to have a child and have exhausted all other avenues for conceiving a child of their own. But many of these techniques raise major moral questions and can create thorny legal dilemmas that are presented to our courts for resolution.

*Reproductive technologies* is a very broad term that refers to medications given women to stimulate egg production with no intention of egg retrieval; the handling of sperm, such as for insemination; and "assisted reproductive technologies" (ART). Here are a few definitions to begin this process; these are listed in alphabetical order

### U.S. PIONEER REFLECTS ON FUTURE OF ART
(Assisted Reproductive Technology)

Dr. Howard W. Jones Jr. and his wife, Dr. Georgeanna Seegar Jones, helped create the first test tube baby born in the United States. The Joneses are also known for having opened the first in vitro fertilization clinic in America. With the combination of much experience in the field of assisted reproductive technology and good foresight, Dr. Howard Jones recognized a need for an ethics committee early in his career. In 1984 an ethics committee began under the American Fertility Society, known today as the American Society for Reproductive Medicine. Despite the creation of an ethics committee, Dr. Howard Jones recognizes the spirit of commercialization prevalent among doctors today. He adds that while commercialization isn't unique to this field of medicine, it is a disappointment; in the "early days" doctors helped one another.

Source: Randi Hutter Epstein, "Pioneer Reflects on Future of Reproductive Medicine," *The New York Times*, March 22, 2010, NYTimes.com.

for the sake of convenience. The ethical ramifications of each will be discussed in the following chapters.

*ART*—In this book, ART will be restricted as per the Centers for Disease Control and Prevention (CDC) definition.[2] ART refers to fertility treatments that involve the handling of both eggs and sperm. Usually, this entails drug-induced stimulation of egg maturation and release, followed by the surgical removal of a woman's eggs from her ovaries. The eggs are combined with sperm in a petri dish in the laboratory for fertilization to take place, and the resulting embryos are implanted in the woman's uterus. There are several variations of this procedure, and these will be explained further in this and succeeding chapters.

*ART Cycle*—(or simply, **cycle**) refers to the hormonal preparation of the woman with fertility drugs, harvesting or retrieval of the mature eggs, fertilization, and transfer of the embryos into the woman's uterus. The cycle may result in a pregnancy, or something may interrupt it in any of these steps along the way. In this book, "cycle" refers to the ART cycle only, unless otherwise specified.

*Days*—In terms of the embryos created through in vitro fertilization: Day 0 is the day the egg is fertilized with the sperm in the laboratory. Day 1 is the first day AFTER the egg is fertilized. These fertilized eggs, or zygotes, can be frozen on Day 1, Day 3, or Day 5.

*Donor Insemination (DI)*—Sperm is procured, usually by masturbation, from a man who is not the legal father of the child. There are differences, in terms of maternal health-related risk, between fresh and frozen sperm samples. The sperm is used to inseminate the woman through placing it in her uterus (IUI) or fallopian tube (GIFT), or to fertilize eggs in a petri dish in the laboratory.

*Egg Donation*—Eggs are procured from reproductive-age females who have received drugs to stimulate egg production. These eggs are fertilized with sperm in the laboratory, or (more rarely) placed into the woman's fallopian tube through a laparoscope.

*Embryo*—This term denotes a human being from conception (when a human egg is fertilized by human sperm) until eight weeks gestation. There are some other terms for certain stages of the embryo that may be familiar: when sperm fertilizes an egg, a fertilized egg or **zygote** is produced. At five–seven days post-fertilization, the name given to the microscopic human is **blastocyst**.

*Embryo Adoption*—A couple who are not the genetic parents of the embryo are given the embryo of and by another couple: this is not a legal adoption, per se. It requires hormonal preparation of the recipient mother, and an embryo transfer.

*Embryo Transfer*—The movement of an embryo from a petri dish or other container in the lab through the woman's cervix into her uterus. This can be a previously frozen or a so-called fresh embryo; hormonal preparation of the recipient is required.

*Fertility Drugs*—refers to any of several medications that promote egg maturation and release from the ovaries; while some are oral medications, most of these are injectable. They are used in all the assisted reproductive technologies, and result in some level of ovarian hyperstimulation.

*Fetus*—This is the name of the developing human, from the end of the eighth week following conception until birth.

*Gamete*—refers to either the sperm or egg (ovum).

*Gamete Intrafallopian Transfer (GIFT)*—The woman's eggs are surgically removed (after stimulation by fertility drugs) and, with the sperm, are inserted into the fallopian tubes, where fertilization normally occurs. This is a laparoscopic procedure.

*Intracytoplasmic Sperm Injection (ICSI)*—usually a procedure for male infertility, a single sperm is injected into an egg in this laboratory procedure. An egg, harvested from a woman, is placed under the microscope and held in place. A small hole is made in the egg's membrane. A single sperm, prepared by having a portion of its tail removed, is placed into the egg using specialized equipment. If the egg is successfully fertilized, the resulting embryo is placed into the woman's womb (uterus), which has been hormonally prepared to receive it.

*Intrauterine Insemination (IUI)*—Sperm, from a husband or donor, is placed in a woman's uterus via a catheter in this procedure.

*In Vitro Fertilization (IVF)*—A procedure in which eggs, matured through use of fertility medications, are laparoscopically removed from a woman and mixed with sperm from a man, and the resulting embryo(s) is/are placed into the woman's uterus through the cervix.

*Laparoscopic; laparoscopically*—A surgical procedure in which one or more small incisions are made in the abdomen to allow the insertion of instruments, including a camera, which is part of the viewing apparatus (a laparoscope). The laparoscope is attached to a video monitor, so the surgeon can see the inside of the abdomen and pelvis, and perform procedures without "opening" the abdomen.

*Preimplantation Genetic Diagnosis (PGD)*—This testing of IVF embryos uses one or more cells from an early embryo to check for inherited conditions/diseases/abnormal chromosomes. Following the outcome of the testing, usually only unaffected embryos are implanted in the woman's uterus.

*Prenatal Genetic Testing*—testing of the blood of a pregnant woman or the amniotic fluid or placental tissue of the developing child for inherited and/or chromosomal abnormalities.

*Surrogacy*—the gestating (carrying in the womb) of a child by a woman who will not act as the mother who rears the child.

    *Altruistic Surrogacy*—a woman who gestates a child for another without payment.

    *Commercial Surrogacy*—a woman who is paid to gestate a child for someone else.

    *Genetic Surrogacy*—The woman who gestates the child also contributes the egg, so she is the genetic mother of the child.

    *Gestational Surrogacy*—a woman who carries to term a child for another; she does not provide the egg. Genetic and gestational surrogacy may be either commercial or altruistic.

*Zygote*—a newly fertilized egg.

## BIRTH RATES IN WOMEN OVER FORTY

Marilyn Nolen used assisted reproductive therapy (ART) to give birth to twins at the age of fifty-five. Nolen is just one of many women who are using ARTs to have children past the age of forty. The number of pregnant women ages 40–44 increased 4 percent in 2008. Also, pregnant women past the age of forty were more likely to be first-time mothers than not. However, doctors warn that women should not be misled into thinking postponing pregnancy is always a good option. There is only a 10 percent chance that a woman after the age of forty can conceive naturally, and having children later in life has an increased risk of medical complications for the mother, including gestational diabetes and hypertension during pregnancy.

Source: Courtney Hutchison, "Birth Rates Rise Among Women Over 40, CDC Finds," ABC News Medical Unit, April 7, 2010, abcnews.go.com.

*Zygote Intrafallopian Transfer (ZIFT)*—An IVF embryo is placed into a woman's fallopian tube through a laparoscope.

Of the entities listed above, these involve primarily medical intervention into natural reproductive processes: fertility drugs, IUI, GIFT, ZIFT, IVF, and ICSI. A second group of these technologies goes further and requires participation of another person in order to achieve conception and/or birth: donor insemination (DI), egg donation, and surrogate motherhood.[3] In some cases, the genetic material of the third party is required, and in others, such as gestational surrogacy, it is not.

From a theological perspective, reproductive technologies—the ones that do not involve third party contributors and those that do—raise ethical issues. These issues are associated with one's understanding of the theology of the family related to reproduction that is outlined in Scripture and Christian tradition. For example, Roman Catholic tradition, based on natural law, has taught that most interventions in the reproductive process are immoral because they interfere with the natural order of creation (and procreation) that God has ordained.[4] Others allow for technological intervention but do not allow any third parties into the process. We will evaluate both groups of reproductive technologies from the perspective of the biblical teaching on the family.

## Is Infertility on the Rise?

Infertility statistics are not easily accessed. The Centers for Disease Control and Prevention (CDC) found that, by 2002, the number of women ages 15–44 who had ever utilized infertility services was 7.3 million in the United States alone.[5] The American Society for Reproductive Medicine stated in 2003 that one in seven couples has difficulty conceiving. About 35 percent of infertility stems from tubal difficulties of the female: open and functioning fallopian tubes are necessary for conception to occur. Males contribute or are the source of infertility in approximately 40 percent of the cases. Between 5–10 percent of infertility has no obvious cause.[6]

One of the causes of infertility is a woman's blocked or scarred fallopian tubes. This afflicts 18 percent of infertile couples seeking reproductive technologies. There are various reasons for such scarring; the primary one is sexually transmitted diseases, especially chlamydia. Annually, over one million cases of chlamydia infection are reported to the CDC. Early diagnosis and treatment are very important.[7] Note, however, this accounts at least partially for only 18 percent of cases of infertility. That means that 82 percent—the vast majority—have other causes.

---

### BIG SISTER WITH HER SIBLINGS

At the Care Fertility clinic in Nottingham, Shane and Helen Baxter successfully underwent in vitro fertilization. Helen had two fertilized embryos implanted; one took hold and the couple bore daughter Alice Baxter in 2007. Several years later the couple implanted the remaining three embryos from the in vitro fertilization process. All three embryos took hold and the Baxters now have four children from in vitro fertilization: three infants and one three year old.

Source: Lucy Laing, "Pictured: The Toddler Sister and Her Baby Siblings . . .Who Are Actually Quadruplets," *Mail Online*, March 4, 2010, Dailymail.co.uk.

---

Many techniques have been added to the armamentarium of infertility specialists since the world's first test-tube baby was born in 1978. The numbers of IVF cycles have steadily increased. Analysis of worldwide data lags substantially behind the reporting thereof: the data from 2002 were not published until 2009. In 2002, worldwide there were estimated 601,243 IVF cycles, with a total of 148,208 babies born. This represented a 25 percent increase in the number of IVF cycles over the year 2000.[8]

Data for assisted reproductive technologies in the United States are reported to the Centers for Disease Control and Prevention (http://www.cdc.gov/ART/index.htm). The various procedures and their success rates are published by the Society for Assisted Reproductive

Technology, SART (www.sart.org/). The first IVF baby in the United States was born in 1982, and the most recent available data are from the year 2008. In that year, in the United States, 140,795 cycles were reported. Greater than 99 percent of those were IVF cycles; less than 1 percent of the cycles were either GIFT or ZIFT. Almost all of the cycles included ovarian hyperstimulation, and 64 percent of the cycles included intracytoplasmic sperm injection (ICSI).[9]

## *When ARTs May Be Sought*

These new technologies make a wide variety of reproductive arrangements possible for couples and single persons today. Some of them have become almost routine treatments for infertility while others really present novel ways of having a child. Here is a sample of the ways procreation can occur through these new medical technologies:

- A couple has had three pregnancy losses, and two children who have died before the age of nine months from congenital disorders. They yearn to have a child of their own, but are reluctant to try again. Recently they heard about embryo adoption, and wonder if that may be an option.

- A woman is able to produce eggs but is unable to carry a child to term. She and her husband want to "rent the womb" of another woman to gestate the embryo that will be formed by laboratory fertilization of the wife's egg by the husband's sperm. Is this reasonable? What considerations should be made regarding surrogacy?

- A married couple desires to have a child but the woman wants to avoid any interruption in her career for pregnancy, so her sister offers to carry the child for her. The wife accepts, and the child is born successfully. How does the sister feel about this niece or nephew? What/when do the parents tell the child about their desire for him/her?

- A lesbian couple wants to have a child. One of the women provides the egg, and after it is fertilized by donor sperm, the embryo is implanted in the uterus of her partner. Five years later, they go their separate ways. What happens to the child?

- A couple desiring to have children cannot produce any of the sperm or eggs necessary for conception. So the woman's sister will donate the egg and the man's brother will donate the sperm. Fertilization will occur in vitro, that is, outside the womb, and the embryo will be transferred to the wife of the couple, who will carry the child. Whose names go on the birth certificate? How will the child learn of his/her genetic origins? Is this adultery?

- Two homosexual males want to rear a child. To do so, one man's female friend donates the egg and the other man donates the sperm (or it could even be a mixture of both of their sperm). Another woman is hired to carry the child. What happens if the gestational surrogate refuses to hand over the child?

- A postmenopausal woman in her early sixties with grown children wants to have another child. She is given a donated egg, has it fertilized by donor sperm, and the embryo is implanted in her body for her to carry and give birth to the child. Should this be disallowed by law? How old is too old to have a child? Who pays for the procedure?

- A young man dies tragically, leaving only his mother to mourn his death. She has his sperm posthumously harvested, and recruits a surrogate to supply both the egg and the womb, planning to rear her own grandchild. Who controls the gametes of the dead? Should we allow posthumous gamete retrieval?

- A couple had twins through IVF, and froze five embryos from that cycle. These were implanted two years later, and three of them were

> ## THE LGBT BABY BOOM
>
> Of all the new ways to procreate children available to married couples, it is actually gay/lesbian couples who are some of the primary customers of the infertility industry today. UC Berkeley Professor Charis Thompson calls this the "LGBT baby boom" and estimates that in the San Francisco-based Pacific Reproductive Services, that 85–90 percent of the clients are gay/lesbian. Gay men use surrogates and lesbian women utilize donor insemination to have children.
>
> Source: C. W. Nevius, "More Lesbian Women Becoming Moms," *San Francisco Chronicle*, May 8, 2010: C1, sfgate.com.

born. Technically, these three are the rest of a set of quintuplets. What do the parents tell these children?

• A fertility clinic has four thousand embryos left in frozen storage. The staff has tried without success to contact the persons whose embryos these are. What should they do with them?

## *The Infertility Industry*

Debora L. Spar, a business administration professor at Harvard, wrote an excellent tome, *The Baby Business*. In it, she describes the markets that surround the procuring of babies—through reproductive technologies as well as adoption. She calculated the U.S. market for fertility treatment:

• In 2002, revenue in U.S. dollars for IVF was $1,038,528,000.
• In 2004, fertility drugs alone totaled $1,331,860,000.
• Money spent for gametes in 2004: sperm, $74,380,000; donor eggs, $37,773,000.[10]

Prices of cycles (see page 24) vary, based on maternal age and the procedures done. An average cycle costs more than $12,000 currently.[11]

Spar explains the infertility industry in these words: "There are very few restrictions on fertility treatments and little regulation of providers. . . . The market for fertility in the United States is vibrant, competitive, and expanding in the absence of any kind of formal controls."[12]

## Overview of the Book

In assessing the morality of each of these reproductive technologies, we must first lay some foundational groundwork. We will examine a theology of the family related to reproduction that will set some of the main parameters for the Christian couple (chapter 2). We will use this to evaluate the Roman Catholic prohibition of most reproductive technologies based on the notion of natural law (chapter 3). We will discuss the question of the personhood of the fetus and embryo (chapter 4). If embryos and fetuses are persons from the moment of conception, then that affects the morality of some of these reproductive technologies.

In part II, we will look at the specific reproductive technologies that are being used today. We will take up both artificial insemination and egg donation in chapter 5. IVF, GIFT, and ZIFT are addressed together since they have a number of features in common (chapter 6). Surrogate motherhood is more controversial both in Christian and

---

**THE BUSINESS OF BABY MAKING**

An ad by the Destination Health Exhibition in London advertised the high demands of IVF fertility treatment. The exhibition provided IVF clinics with the opportunity to advertise their services to potential patients from local and abroad locations. The advertisement emphasized the notion that patients attend the exhibition "with money to spend" and they are "eager and willing to spend money on their needs." Overall the ad sounded more like an exhibition for businesses looking to get ahead of the competition than a medical practice looking to treat patients in need.

Source: Michael Cook, "The Lucrative Business of Baby-Making," *BioEdge*, March 30, 2010, Bioedge.org.

secular circles and we will explore its complex issues in chapter 7. We will address prenatal genetic testing and preimplantation genetic diagnosis in chapter 8.

Though we have tried to make the book accessible to someone with little background in this arena, the issues that we will address together are very complex; it would be a disservice to deal with them simplistically. We have attempted to make the medical terminology understandable. Although the moral discussion of these technologies presumes no formal background in ethics, our intent is to do justice to the moral complexity of these issues. This is likely the level that the professional and the more advanced student in this area desire. A few of the chapters (chapters 2–4, particularly) are aimed specifically at the person who has considered these issues before, yet a careful reading of these should prove beneficial to all readers.

*We must think through what the Bible has to say about marriage and family.*

# CHAPTER TWO

# Theology of Family and Procreation

A visit to a city park or playground will reveal many different kinds of families—couples, couples with children, single parents with children, grandparents rearing grandchildren, foster parents with foster children, blended families, and children adopted by single parents or couples, to name a few.

Assisted reproductive technologies have made possible births to infertile couples as well as couples whose gametes are of the same sex, and single persons of either sex. While some think that rearing children is a job for a village, others have competing views.

Is there a biblical blueprint for a family? If so, what is it?

## *Different Types of Families in the Bible*

A survey of Scripture reveals a variety of families. Adam and Eve "begat" Cain and Abel, the former ultimately murdering the latter. Then Cain had to leave his family and live among other people, while Adam and Eve had more children.

Generations later, Abraham was impatient for God to give him children, so he acquiesced to Sarah's plan of fathering a child by her servant Hagar—the first known surrogate. Later, when their physical bodies seemed beyond hope of procreating, Abraham and Sarah had a child, Isaac: the promised one.

Isaac and Rebekah had twins that sired markedly different nations. The younger, Jacob, had children with his wives as well as his wives' servants, and had twelve sons and one daughter as a result. And all these families are included in the first thirty chapters of Genesis!

Fast-forward to the New Testament. Elizabeth and Zechariah, both advanced in age, became parents of John the Baptist. Mary, mother of Jesus, was initially an unwed pregnant young girl, who has rightly been honored for centuries for her faithfulness to her Lord. Later, when He hung on the cross, Jesus presented His mother to His disciple John, who would be her caretaker from that point onward (John 19:26–27).

### NEW DEFINITIONS OF FAMILY?

In her HBO documentary, "A Family Is a Family Is a Family: A Rosie O'Donnell Celebration," Rosie O'Donnell promotes her views on gay marriage equality. A large portion of the movie is composed of children's testimonies about living in a family with gay parents. O'Donnell uses songs and cartoons to promote same-sex parents and introduce topics like in vitro fertilization, including a scene with sperm dancing and singing to a Frank Sinatra song. While some reviews acclaim the documentary for the positive promotion of gay marriage, others found it fake and uninformative. O'Donnell hopes that the documentary will be shown in schools and lead to classroom discussions about families.

Source: Brent Bozell, "A Rosie O'Donnell Indoctrination," Feb. 12, 2010, Townhall.com.

In addition, the New Testament uses the family metaphor to describe the church (Gal. 6:10; Eph. 2:19). This is consistent with Jesus' statements that His family includes all those who do the will of God (Matt. 12:48–50). With all of these examples and many more recorded in Scripture, can we find a discernible plan for families in the Bible? Or is the structure of the family a cultural construct that can change as social conditions change?

## Creation and Procreation in the Culture of Old Testament Times

Our goal in this chapter is to clarify the teaching of the Bible on the subject of procreation, and apply it to the use of reproductive technologies (particularly the ones that involve collaborating with gamete donors or surrogates). To do this we must think through what the Bible has to say about marriage and the family, though a full-orbed theology of the family is well beyond what is necessary for our present discussion.

Issues related to gender relations, sexuality, and parenting have driven most of the theologically oriented discussion of the family; the bearing of family structure on reproduction has been less frequently explored.[1] The obvious exception to this is in Roman Catholic circles, where procreation has been addressed in great detail from the perspective of natural law. We will take up the Catholic discussion in chapter 3.

### *The Foundation of Sex and Procreation*

From the opening pages of Scripture, marriage, sexuality, and procreation are important themes. The complementary accounts in Genesis 1 and 2 are widely considered a central text that sets the trajectory for the relationship between man and woman in marriage, and the expression of the marital bond in sex and procreation. These chapters establish a critical link between the man and woman in the context of marriage and the procreation of children. The institution of marriage is clearly related to the command in Genesis 1:27 to "be fruitful and multiply."

The creation accounts in Genesis 1 and 2 are complementary, not contradictory, to each other. Genesis 1 provides the broad panoramic overview of creation. Genesis 2 examines the most important aspects of creation, the creation of man and woman, and their relationship to each other and to God, in more detail. The account of the creation of man and woman that is described in Genesis 2:18–25 actually fits into the broader overview of Genesis 1. To be specific, it occurs after the divine initiative in 1:26 to create mankind, and prior to the command to the newly formed couple in 1:28 to begin procreating and populating the earth. Thus, Genesis 1:26 describes generally the creation of humankind, and Genesis 2:18–25 describes specifically the male and female of the species. The first command given them that is recorded by Scripture is the command to procreate (in 1:28).

We believe Genesis 1–2 marks the institution of marriage as one of the creation mandates[2] for several reasons. First, the way that this text is quoted in other places in the New Testament makes it clear that it was originally intended for married couples (Matt. 19:5; Eph. 5:32). Second, the term "leave" is used to suggest that, against common ancient Near Eastern cultural practice in which the bride moved in with the groom and his family, a man and woman who will be intimately related (as the term "cleave" suggests) are to separate emotionally from their families of origin and begin a new family unit of their own.[3] Third, the concept of one flesh clearly involves a sexual unity, though it is not limited to that. Throughout Scripture, it is evident that sexual relations are restricted to the setting of marriage. Thus it seems that Genesis 2:24 is the place where marriage as a divine institution begins.

### Framework for Sex and Procreation

Though it is true that Adam and Eve are representative in a broader sense of the first male and female of the species, it is also true that they set the precedent for heterosexual marriage and for procreation within that setting. The account clearly does not suggest that every male and female must be joined in marriage, but it does indicate that marriage is to be between male and female, and only in marriage is procreation to occur. In other words, in Genesis 1–2, *God designed permanent, monogamous, heterosexual marriage as the sacred context for both sex and procreation.* We see continuity between God's creation of the family in Genesis 1–2 and the command to procreate within that context. This ideal of the family seems to be basic to God's creative design, however extended the family became due to cultural and economic factors.

### Safeguarding the Genesis Ideal

However, the creation account does not mandate such close continuity between sexual intercourse and procreation. One could argue that certainly Scripture did not anticipate nor address the complex methods of reproduction that are in use today. In addition, the perspective of the creation account on sexual relations must be balanced by other parts of Scripture that extend the purpose of sexual relations beyond procreation alone, though we would insist that procreation is the unique end of both marriage and sex.[4]

Certainly sex is reserved for marriage, but simply because the creation account links marriage and procreation, it does not follow that procreation must always follow from marital sexual relations. The notion of one flesh, though it certainly involves physical intimacy, goes beyond the physical alone, and includes emotional and spiritual unity as well. Marriage is to be characterized by oneness between the partners, of which the physical is a part. The teaching of the creation account is that procreation is to take place within the oneness of a total marriage relationship, not necessarily a specific instance of sexual intercourse.

Portions of Old Testament law were designed to safeguard this Genesis ideal of the family. The prohibitions against illicit sexual relations assumed the background of Genesis 1–2, and functioned to preserve the family from breakdown. The sexual prohibitions/laws in Leviticus 18 prohibit sexual relationships that deviate from what was sanctioned in Genesis 1–2, i.e., sex between a heterosexual couple in marriage. Incest, homosexuality, adultery (specifically cultic prostitution), and premarital sex are considered outside God's design and thus prohibited.

Though the list of deviations from the Genesis ideal is not exhaustive and gives no specific reason for these prohibitions, it seems obvious that these violate the ideal for marriage and sexuality that is rooted in the Genesis account of creation. Keeping the creation ideal intact and free from influences that would undermine it was considered central to the preservation of Israel as a society set apart as God's holy nation (Ex. 19:6), particularly since sexual purity and the purity of worship were seen as closely interrelated. What this suggests is that the Levitical sexual prohibitions/laws treat the Genesis ideal for marriage and sexuality as a norm, and violations of the norm were taken very seriously.

In addition, parts of the Wisdom Literature presuppose that the Genesis account is a norm for monogamy when the Proverbs urge faithfulness to one's wife as a moral imperative (Prov. 5:15–20; also Eccl. 9:9). More significantly, the prophets clearly assume the Genesis norm of monogamy when they compare Israel's exclusive relationship with God to a faithful, monogamous marriage (Ezek. 16:1–22; Hos. 2:1, 19–20; Mal. 2:10–16).[5] This concept is echoed in the New Testament with the figure of speech of the church as the permanent, monogamous bride of Christ (Eph. 5:22–31).

### Genesis Affirmed by Jesus and Paul

This treatment of the Genesis ideal is echoed in the New Testament, when in Romans 1:18–32 Paul forbids homosexual sex based on its violation of the natural order of sexuality, derived from the Genesis ideal, which Paul is taking as a norm for heterosexual sex and a prohibition on homosexuality. It is further affirmed by Jesus in His teaching on divorce in Matthew 19:3–9, when He explicitly appeals to Genesis 1–2 as the foundation for His argument prohibiting divorce (except in the case of adultery).

It seems that both Jesus and Paul treat the Genesis account as a bit more than an ideal—but also as a norm that they expected people to follow (though in Matthew 19 Jesus allows for an exception in the event of adultery). Under such a norm, it is important that procreation maintain "the exclusive nature of spousal cooperation."[6] Marriage, then, is "the normative context for the transmission of human life."[7]

## Departures from the Genesis Ideal

### *Ensuring the Family Line*

When it comes to procreation, however, it gets more complicated. A closer reading of the Old Testament reveals some practices that may have constituted departures from the norm, some of which involved novel reproductive arrangements. For example, levirate marriage (Deut. 25:5–10; Ruth 3–4) was employed to continue the lineage of a woman's deceased husband should she be left childless at his death.

This tradition illustrates the general inseparability of marriage and procreation that was characteristic of the ancient world, not just in accounts of people in the Old Testament. In this arrangement, a woman who was widowed and childless could appeal to the closest male next of kin to marry her and father a child who would take over the inheritance rights of his deceased father and take care of his mother as well. The importance of this practice was due to some of the cultural factors governing economic life in the ancient world. First, economic survival depended on access to productive land for farming or grazing purposes. A person who did not have access to land was reduced either to tenant farming or to charity; thus, passing on the inheritance of property to children was critical to the extended family's economic well-being. Second, children were critical economic assets, not only to work the land, but to take care of parents when they became unable to work any longer. Therefore, to be childless was to invite destitution in a couple's later years. This is one of the reasons why Scripture refers to children as a gift (Ps. 127:3 NASB). Third, inheritance rights came through the male, thereby putting childless widows in a particularly vulnerable position. So the law made provision for a childless widow to have a child, to provide an heir to her deceased husband's property, and to ensure her economic security.

### Is Levirate Marriage Comparable to Donor Insemination?

Some suggest that this practice provides a biblical precedent for third party involvement in procreation in a form such as donor insemination.[8] However, levirate marriage is not analogous to third party collaborative reproductive techniques for two reasons. First, there was technically no third party introduced into the reproductive matrix since the childless woman in view was a widow. Her husband was not only being replaced for purposes of reproduction, it was his death that made the entire levirate arrangement necessary. Second, this is not a case of simply inseminating the woman so that she could give birth, with the sperm donor taking no parenting responsibility. The near relative actually married her and took full responsibility for supporting her and the child(ren) who would be born through their union. The requirement that the near relative marry the woman suggests that levirate marriage actually supports the Genesis ideal by keeping procreation within the context of marriage.

However, the child produced by the levirate marriage was not legally the biological father's child. He was the child of his deceased father for purposes of inheritance and property rights. For example, in the first recorded biblical episode of levirate marriage in Genesis 38, Onan refused to impregnate his deceased brother's wife because the child would belong to his brother. God considered it evil for Onan "to keep from producing offspring for his brother" (Gen. 38:9). Though the biological father was responsible for the child and the mother both, the child was not an heir of the biological father but the deceased father.

The near relative would be similar to a sperm donor in one sense, in which the donor is the biological father but under the law does not have paternal rights to the child. Of course, today the donor does not marry the woman he donates to, as in levirate marriage, nor is he responsible for providing for the child, two major differences that finally undermine the analogy with levirate marriage to contemporary sperm donation.

A further complicating factor is that the law that mandates levirate marriage (Deut. 25:5–10) does not specify that the near relative fulfilling the procreative function be unmarried. In fact, more often than not, obedience to this law involved polygamy, which is a violation of the Genesis ideal of monogamous marriage. So the redeemer could be in the interesting position of obeying the law and violating the Genesis ideal for monogamous marriage at the same time. Thus, the levirate marriage arrangement does involve some distance from the Genesis ideal in order to account for harsh economic realities for childless widows.

### Surrogacy in the Old Testament

A second novel reproductive arrangement found in the Old Testament is surrogacy. This appears to have been a widely accepted cultural practice in the ancient Near East and was employed by both Abraham and Jacob in the patriarchal narratives (Gen. 16, 30). The reason for surrogacy and its apparently widespread use in the ancient world is similar to the law concerning levirate marriage, due to the close connection between children, and inheritance/property rights. A childless couple was economically vulnerable, particularly in old age, and had no one to pass on their property to when they died. In addition, childlessness in the ancient world was a general source of shame that often created a sense of desperation on behalf of couples, especially women, to employ means outside of marriage in order to have children.

In the Genesis accounts of surrogacy, there is no overt condemnation attached to the use of surrogates to alleviate female infertility. It is merely described in the course of the narratives of the lives of

Abraham and Jacob. However, in Abraham's case with Hagar, it could be argued that the consequences of his going in to Hagar were so negative that that is tantamount to a judgment on the practice. Perhaps God simply allowed the outcome to speak for itself as a negative evaluation of the practice.

That said, the Abraham and Hagar narrative is about more than the use of a surrogate. The far weightier issue is Abraham's and Sarah's lack of trust in God to keep His covenant promise to make their descendents numerous and to make him a great nation. Abraham's role as covenant mediator is a unique case; thus, it is not clear that any normative biblical teaching on third party collaborative reproduction can be deduced.

### Another Patriarch

What about the case of Abraham's grandson Jacob, in his use of surrogates? Though Jacob, too, is a patriarch who carries on the covenant, in his case there is no other issue of faith as was the case with Abraham. The problem is that one of Jacob's two wives is childless. By Genesis 30, Leah has had a number of children, but Rachel has none. Rachel is so grieved that she instructs her maid to have sexual relations with Jacob and she finally ends up with a child, whom she considers completely her own. The maid, acting as a surrogate, would not serve as a mother to the son she has borne.

This would seem to be a case in which surrogacy is accepted as a normal practice, without the obvious and disastrous consequences that accompanied Abraham and Sarah's use of a surrogate. To be fair, however, there was considerable strife between the different women in Jacob's life, which may be a narrative clue that all was not well in the arrangement.

### Surrogacy Then and Now

However, there are some clear differences between surrogacy in the ancient world and surrogacy today. First, surrogacy in ancient times was not a consensual choice of the surrogate, nor was she compensated in any way. In fact, surrogacy was generally practiced with household slaves/maids, who had no choice in the matter and no rights to the children they bore. Slavery and surrogacy were thus closely intertwined, making it quite different from the normal practice of surrogacy today.[9]

A second difference was that in the ancient world, the surrogate was impregnated by sexual intercourse, not by technological means, as is the norm today. It is not clear why surrogacy did not constitute adultery in the ancient world, though it may have had something to do with the status of most surrogates as slaves. It may have been that with maids being considered more akin to property than wives, that sex with maids was in a different category altogether.

### Multiple Wives and Concubines

Polygamy was another practice that was accepted in the ancient world, though one should be careful about exaggerating its extent—it was usually restricted to families with the means to support multiple wives.[10] It also constituted a departure from the Genesis ideal of monogamous marriage yet was practiced by a variety of notable Old Testament patriarchs and kings.

Polygamy was one of the ways to deal with harsh economic realities that came from living in a predominantly agricultural society. It also had a demographic basis as well, since in the ancient world there was generally an imbalance between the number of females to males. Due to the frequency of wars and other military conflicts, men often died prematurely. Given the patriarchal society in the ancient world, women were not generally in a position where self-support was possible—they were most often connected either to their family of origin or to a husband in order to achieve some economic security. In addition, it was not uncommon for women to die in childbirth. This put pressure on the men to have additional wives for childbearing purposes. Given the connection between procreation and prosperity, which made children economic assets, a greater number of children brought additional workers to farm or tend flocks.[11]

A similar pattern to polygamy occurred with concubinage.[12] Concubines were not considered wives in the ancient world, but childbearing was one of the primary roles they fulfilled. It is not considered equivalent to polygamy, since they were not technically married to the men under whose roof and care they lived. They were generally considered of a lower social rank and, similar to polygamy, the practice was restricted to families of some economic means and was often consensual, with the women trading off childbearing for a measure of economic security. The difference between concubines and surrogates is that concubines had a higher status and were closer to being wives than slaves/maids.

## *Divorce*

A final practice that was allowed by God in both testaments is divorce. The Genesis design is that of marriage being permanent, as the notion of "cleaving" or "being united to" one's spouse indicates. In addition, the concept of "two becoming one flesh" strongly suggests that their bond was intended to be permanent. Yet the Old Testament law outlines measures that protect the dignity of women in the case of divorce, by preventing the woman from becoming akin to property that can be repeatedly transferred between husbands (Deut. 24:1–4).

Divorce is acknowledged as inevitable due to the callousness of human beings (Matt. 19:8—Jesus describes this as a concession to their hard hearts), and regulated so that women would not be abused or treated like property. The law functioned as "damage control" in the case of divorce.[13] Jesus clarified the law on divorce, arguing that God's original design was for it to be permanent but allowed for an exception in the case of unfaithfulness (Matt. 19:9). Jesus appealed to the Genesis ideal as a norm governing behavior, which shocked the disciples (Matt. 19:10), but nonetheless allowed for an exception. This suggests that the Genesis ideal was functioning for Jesus as a prima facie norm, not an absolute.

# What Can We Conclude?

Thus, hermeneutically, we are in a complicated position. The Genesis account clearly sets the trajectory for marriage, sexuality, and procreation in the direction of permanent, monogamous marriage as the sacred context for procreation. It demonstrates God's original design for procreation to occur within the exclusive marital bond. The implicit appeal of the sexual prohibitions/laws in Leviticus 18, 20 to the creation account, the presupposition of monogamy in the Wisdom Literature and the Prophets, as well as Paul's and Jesus' use of Genesis 1–2 suggest that the Genesis ideal actually functions as a prima facie norm, though admittedly, it is more of an absolute in the area of sexuality than procreation.

## *Departures from the Ideal*

When it comes to procreation, the Old Testament describes some common practices that constituted departures from the Genesis ideal. Clearly some of these were sin, examples of which include Solomon's taking of numerous foreign wives in order to solidify military alliances (and thereby undercut trust in God for Israel's national security). It is also clear that Abraham and Sarah's use of Hagar as a surrogate was sin—a clear violation of God's explicit command to them to procreate naturally and trust Him with producing the heir to the covenant.

In other cases, the narrative gives the reader some clues that all is not quite right with the arrangement, as is the case with Jacob's use of surrogates. In other examples, it is not as clear. For example, as mentioned earlier, obeying the mandate for levirate marriage could easily put someone into a polygamous situation, and though that does have some distance from the Genesis ideal, it is hard to see how that is sin, since it involved obedience to an explicit command of the law. That would still be the case even though the New Testament clarifies the expectation of monogamy for the church. Further it appears that divorce is not necessarily sin, though it too involves some distance from God's original design that marriage be permanent.

## Cultural Practices and Norms

However, an accepted cultural practice and a moral norm that transcends culture are not synonymous. Simply because surrogacy existed as a practice that was utilized by the patriarchs says very little about its acceptability as a reproductive alternative today, particularly since surrogacy in the ancient world was so different from the type practiced today. For reasons that usually relate to some form of damage control from living in a broken world, God tolerated many practices that were not in accordance with His original design, including some that were not consistent with His creation design for marriage and the family.

As previously mentioned, the biblical teaching on divorce (Deut. 24:1–4; Matt. 19:3–9) is an excellent example. The pattern for marriage in Matthew 19 is clear that it was "from the beginning," a reference to the creation account. The toleration of any of these departures in the patriarchal era does not necessarily legitimate their use today, especially given the connection in the creation account between the context of heterosexual marriage and procreation.

On the other hand, it is significant that the Old Testament tolerated some deviations from God's creation model. It is true that toleration does not establish normative patterns and, indeed, implies a deviation from them.

Conversely, actions that violate the ideal set up at creation were not necessarily morally disallowed, though the restrictions seem to be much tighter with sexuality than with procreation—though not be the best option, they are not prohibited.

Few people view alternative reproductive arrangements made necessary by infertility as the best option. But simply because it is not the best option, fully consistent with the model of creation, it does not follow that it is always morally prohibited. Thus, appeal to the creation ideal, without further argument, may not be sufficient to settle the debate concerning the moral acceptability of third party contributors to the procreative process.

### The New Testament and Genesis

Part of this further argument is found in the manner in which the New Testament writers appealed to the Genesis ideal. In the New Testament, an appeal to the creation ideal to mediate a controversy usually settles the issue. For example, Paul appeals to creation in Romans 1:18–32 to argue that homosexuality goes against God's design for human sexuality established at creation. That is considered the principal argument employed, though he also refers to the negative consequences of deviating from the creation model for sexuality.

Similarly, when dealing with the roles of women in the church and the home (1 Cor. 11:8–9; 1 Tim. 2:11–15), Paul appeals to the model of creation and little else to settle the issue. On the one hand, the Old Testament did not label some deviations from the creation model as sin. But when the New Testament uses the creation model to support its case, there is not much further argument needed nor given.

Therefore, the ideal set up by God's design at creation and the New Testament's appeal to its authority tilts the biblical balance against third party contributors. Thus it seems best to say that Scripture is skeptical about third party contributors to reproduction, without saying that Scripture teaches an absolute prohibition of all such arrangements.

### A Christian Perspective

We would recommend, for a number of reasons that we will spell out in the chapters to come, that Christian couples not pursue third party contributors, but on the basis of Scripture, we are not prepared to call every use of them necessarily sinful.

One example of third party contributors that we would not call necessarily sinful is the use of a surrogate mother in the case of a couple with embryos left over from IVF and without the ability to implant any remaining embryos themselves, due to medical issues such as a hysterectomy. Since the couple wants to raise their genetic children and not discard them (which would be wrong), and there is little point to donating embryos that the couple desires to raise, the best alternative is the use of a surrogate to gestate the remaining embryos currently in storage. Though we can debate the wisdom of creating excess embryos, use of a surrogate may be a form of acceptable damage control to prevent the much more problematic discarding of embryos.

In the consideration of third party contributors to reproduction, an important question arises. Given that marriage and procreation are so entwined, is adoption a violation of it? Adoption is clearly a separation of the biological and social roles of a parent, and is not consistent with the link between marriage and procreation/parenting. *Adoption, however, is not procreation* but, rather, is fundamentally an act of charity, based on the biblical admonitions to care for the fatherless and to love one's neighbor.[14] It is a solution to an unwanted pregnancy or other situation of a parent being unable or unwilling to care for her child.

Adoption can be appropriately viewed as a virtuous "rescue operation" that is centered on the welfare of the child being adopted. Of course, adoption is an intrinsically good act since it is one of the primary figures of speech to describe a person's relationship to God. But the fact that adoption is encouraged as a virtuous act has nothing to do with setting norms for procreation, since they are fundamentally two different things. Nothing necessarily follows from the Bible's teaching on adoption that is relevant to setting parameters on procreation.

In general, reproductive technologies that do not introduce third parties into the exclusivity of the marital relationship can be considered consistent with God's original design that procreation occur within the exclusive setting of permanent, monogamous, heterosexual marriage. Those that enable an infertile couple to conceive using medical technology without third party collaborators can, for the most part, be embraced as morally legitimate. About those that involve a third party contributor, the trajectory of Scripture is established by the norm set up by the Genesis account of marriage and procreation.

*The Catholic Church has been significantly out in front*

*in addressing the reproductive revolution.*

# CHAPTER THREE

# Catholic Natural Law and Procreation

M aria's vision of her doctor was blurred by fresh tears. While "no evidence of abnormality" seemed like good news, it didn't feel like good news. Three years of trying to conceive a baby, and still no success.

What was wrong? Her system seemed to be working well. There was no evidence of abnormality—except the failure to conceive. What were they going to do now? Maria was brought up in a staunchly Catholic family; Alex, in a home slightly less so. They both wanted to honor God in their lives. So what were their choices now? Listening to Dr. Davis explain her options, Maria knew she and Alex would need to talk with their priest. And maybe they could get to know that new family in their church—the fortyish couple who were parents to a toddler.

Maria and Alex consoled one another—again—that night, and they discussed their next step. The following morning, Maria telephoned Father Joseph's office and made an appointment. He could see them on Friday of that week.

## Robin's Story

On Thursday, as Maria was grocery shopping, she bumped into Robin, the forty-something woman, with her toddler. Robin recognized Maria, and introduced her to two-year-old Charlie, who was squirming in the grocery cart seat. Maria commented about Charlie's energy, and Robin said that he had turned her life upside down.

"How so?" asked Maria.

"Well, Bruce and I struggled for over ten years to get pregnant, and then, suddenly, here was Charlie!"

Maria's attention was riveted on Robin's words. "How did it happen?"

"It's a long story. If you really want to hear about it, we'd need to sit down and talk for a while. But have you ever heard of egg donation?"

Charlie, not interested in hearing any more adult conversation, loudly made his frustration known. "I have to go—time for Charlie's lunch." With that, Robin headed toward the checkout.

Yes, Maria had heard of egg donation. But she didn't know what exactly she thought of it. Was it a reasonable thing to do? She would have to think more about this, and ask Father Joseph about it when they met the next day.

## A Talk with Their Priest

Alex and Maria had moved to their new home and parish about three years ago, and thus did not know Father Joseph well. He spent the bulk of their meeting the next day getting to know them. He talked with them about the time they had spent getting to know each other before their marriage, and the detailed plans they had made for the wedding.

He talked in general about how the Catholic Church views marriage and procreation. They were disappointed to realize that a quick fix did not await them, but also recognized that such important, weighty decisions as they were making need ample consideration. They agreed to meet with him over the next several weeks in order to discuss these matters further.

During the ensuing meetings, Father Joseph guided them through three important documents that speak to marriage and family, and finally, reproductive technologies in particular. He invited their questions, and asked some himself.

## *Roman Catholicism's Reasoning*

Maria and Alex are part of the faith tradition that has produced the vast majority of the religiously based discussion of reproductive technologies.[1] Catholic theology traditionally has had a great interest in bioethics and particularly in the values expressed in procreation.

Early on, the Catholic Church spoke out against contraception. Its application of Catholic tradition to the development of numerous artificial methods of birth control, including abortion, made for a ready transition to the discussion on reproductive interventions. Thus, Roman Catholicism was well situated to respond to the variety of reproductive technological developments of recent years. As a result, the Catholic Church has been significantly out in front of other religious traditions in addressing the reproductive revolution, and has much to teach Christians in other faith traditions.

The Catholic tradition based on natural law has emphasized the strict continuity between sex in marriage, procreation, and parenthood. According to natural law, in the process of procreation, if everything progresses as God originally designed it, sexual relations result in conception and childbirth. In the same way that God designed an acorn to grow into an oak tree, He designed sexual relations by nature to come to fruition in the birth of a child. Thus there is a God-ordained, natural continuity between sex in marriage and parenthood.

Every sexual encounter has the potential for conception, and every conception has the potential for childbirth and parenthood. This is why sex is reserved for marriage, and why Catholic tradition makes little room for any reproductive technology that would interfere with a natural process that is the result of creation. It also rules out any third party involvement that would replace one of the partners in the married couple. Only with husband and wife in heterosexual marriage is it morally legitimate to procreate children.

Further, there is a natural and fundamental unity between sexual relations and procreation. Procreation cannot occur apart from marital sexual intercourse, and every conjugal act in marriage must be open to procreation as the natural result of God's creation design.[2] Since intercourse has as its intended end the procreation of children, any action such as birth control that prevents it from achieving that end is not allowed. Thus in every sexual act, husband and wife must be open to procreation, and cannot do anything that would break the structural unity of that act of sexual intercourse.

By employing contraception and/or abortion, sex is divorced from its procreative purpose. And by introducing assisted reproduction, procreation is separated from its essential roots in sexual intercourse. For the couple committed to Catholic tradition, this leaves few options for them to procreate other than through normal sexual relations, as Father Joseph explained to Maria and Alex.

He referred to three official Vatican documents as the bases for the Catholic Church's teaching on procreation: the *Humanae Vitae*, the *Donum Vitae*, and the *Dignitas Personae*. These documents are briefly summarized below.

## Humanae Vitae

Pope Paul VI issued the *Humanae Vitae: On the Regulation of Birth* on July 25, 1968. (Ironically on the tenth anniversary of this encyclical, Louise Brown, the first test-tube baby, was born in England.) The pope was taking aim at the rise of contraception, and this work is considered the foundational modern philosophical and theological contribution to Catholic reproductive ethics.

The general tenor of the encyclical is that "Marriage and conjugal love are *by their nature* [emphasis added] ordained toward the begetting and educating of children. Children are really the supreme gift of marriage and contribute very substantially to the welfare of the parents."[3] That is, God ordained marriage for the procreation of children.

Here is the crux of the Church's argument. When God designed sexual relations, He invested the action with two inseparable meanings: the *unitive* and the *procreative*. The unitive aspect enables husband and wife to experience the oneness of marriage; the procreative, to transmit life to the next generation, reflecting the creative hand of God. Both are essential to sex in marriage and cannot be separated. Thus, contraception is judged a moral evil because it keeps the procreative side of the act from being fulfilled. The encyclical puts it this way:

> That teaching [that every sexual act must be open to procreation], is founded upon the inseparable connection, willed by God and unable to be broken by man on his own initiative, between the two meanings of the conjugal act: the unitive meaning and the procreative meaning. Indeed, by its intimate structure, the conjugal act, while most closely uniting husband and wife, capacitates them for the generation of new lives, according to laws inscribed in the very being of man and of woman. By safeguarding both these essential aspects, the unitive and the procreative, the conjugal act preserves in its fullness the sense of true mutual love and its ordination towards man's most high calling to parenthood.[4]

This statement, foundational to official Catholic teaching on reproduction, lays out the primary tenet that individual husbands and wives must not intentionally separate the two divinely ordained and essential structural elements of sex in marriage. These two elements are rooted in the nature of human beings, and ultimately in the will of God who placed that nature in them.

The encyclical states, "To use this divine gift [of sex in marriage] destroying, if only partially, its meaning and purpose [by separating the unitive and procreative] is to contradict the nature of both man and woman and of their most intimate relationship, and therefore it is to contradict the plan of God and His will."[5] Thus it is based on natural law because the teaching is grounded in that which is natural for human beings and the natural process, both of which are natural because they are ordained by God.

Contraception, sterilization (unless medically necessary), and elective abortion are all prohibited by the teaching of this encyclical.

## BIOETHICS AND NATURAL LAW

In February of 2010 Pope Benedict XVI argued that a proper system of bioethics accounts for human dignity, and hence requires the use of natural law. The pope asserted that just as God loves every individual in a unique way, we are called to love and value persons. And just as God affirms the human dignity of all persons, bioethics must incorporate human dignity. A good system of ethics demands universal principles that provide a common denominator for all of humanity, one that recognizes human life is intrinsically valuable from its first moment to its end and one that recognizes that human life is an inalienable subject of rights that must never be neglected. Further, the pope warned that we must recognize the potential danger of a legislation that leads to a relativistic drift of ethics. He concluded that natural moral law allows humanity to avoid such a danger; it provides a system that values both humans and all of creation.

Source: "Pontiff: Bioethics Needs Natural Law," Global Zenit News, February 14, 2010, zenit.org.

## Donum Vitae

A second influential Vatican document was issued on February 22, 1987. It is called the "Instruction of Respect for Human Life in Its Origin and on the Dignity of Procreation,"[6] but often referred to as *Donum Vitae*.

The Instruction acknowledges that science and technology are a significant expression of the dominion that God originally entrusted to mankind at creation, of which medicine in general is a significant part. But technology cannot be exempt from moral assessment: moral principles from natural law serve to limit technology appropriately.[7]

The fundamental values that limit the application of reproductive technology are twofold: "the life of the human being called into existence and the special nature of the transmission of human life in marriage."[8] The first of these values has to do with the moral status of the embryo (and fetus, by extension) and the concern to protect embryos from the moment of conception. The Instruction goes into great depth in discussing the embryo's right to life from conception until death. It addresses questions about prenatal diagnosis, research and experimentation on embryos, and the use of embryos in reproductive technologies such as in vitro fertilization. In general, reproductive methods that involve intentional destruction of embryonic life are not morally allowed.

The second fundamental value related to assisted reproduction is "the special nature of the transmission of human life in marriage." Here the Instruction reaffirms the essential teaching of *Humanae Vitae* and states that "from the moral point of view a truly responsible procreation vis-à-vis the unborn child must be the fruit of marriage. . . . The fidelity of the spouses in the unity of marriage involves reciprocal respect of their right to become a father and a mother only through each other. . . . In marriage and in its indissoluble unity [is] the only setting worthy of truly responsible procreation."[9]

Therefore, any reproductive interventions that involve third party genetic or gestational contributors would not be allowed.[10] The Instruction insists that these interventions violate the reciprocal commitment between the spouses in marriage; violate the right of the child; can hinder developing personal identity; and potentially damage the stability of the family for society.[11] The only reproductive technologies that are possible for faithful Catholic couples are those that use the genetic material of husband and wife. Artificial insemination by donor (AID), egg donation, and surrogate motherhood are not consistent with Catholic teaching.

The *Donum Vitae* evaluates reproductive technologies that do not involve third party contributors. In answer to the question "What connection is required from the moral point of view between procreation and the conjugal act?" the Instruction quotes the central point of *Humanae Vitae*,[12] then further specifies and clarifies this central tenet of Catholic teaching. It states that "the same doctrine concerning the link between the meanings of the conjugal act and between the goods of marriage throws light on the moral problem of homologous artificial fertilization, *since it is never permitted to separate these different aspects to such a degree as positively to exclude either the procreative intention or the conjugal act.*"[13]

Thus the only morally legitimate way for fertilization to occur is between husband and wife in marriage and as a result of a specific act of intercourse. The intrinsic nature of the act of sex is rendered incomplete by separating sexual relations from procreation. The Instruction puts it this way:

> From the moral point of view, procreation is deprived of its proper perfection when it is not desired as the fruit of the conjugal act, that is to say, of the specific act of the spouses' union. ... The moral relevance of the link between the meaning of the conjugal act and the goods of marriage as well as the unity of the human being and the dignity of his origin, demand that the procreation of a human person be brought about as the fruit of the conjugal act specific to the love between spouses. [14]

For Catholic teaching, there is no significant moral difference between birth control and reproductive technologies. Each isolates one aspect of sex in marriage: birth control, the unitive aspect; reproductive technologies, the procreative. That is, reproductive interventions stand alone in the discussion—they are not justified by the good consequences (the birth of a child) that may result.

The problem is that the inherent nature of the sex act is violated. With in vitro fertilization, for example, the Instruction states that "the generation of the human person is objectively deprived of its proper perfection: namely that of being the result and fruit of a conjugal act in which the spouses can become cooperators with God for giving life to a new person. The act of conjugal love is considered in the teaching of the Church as the only setting worthy of human procreation."[15] Therefore, in vitro fertilization (IVF), zygote intrafallopian transfer (ZIFT), and intrauterine insemination (IUI) are all judged to be morally problematic.

The Instruction does make an important distinction between a technology that *assists* normal intercourse and one that *replaces* it in the process of trying to conceive a child. Anything that assists intercourse, such as fertility drugs that enable a woman to ovulate regularly, is considered a part of God's wisdom that can be utilized in reproduction. The important aspect is that the unity of sex and procreation is maintained.

What this means more specifically is that conception must occur according to its intended design. The movement of genetic materials may be assisted, but use of technology may not replace normal intercourse. For example, fertilization must always occur inside the body, and masturbation may not be used as a substitute for sex in order to collect sperm outside the body to be reinserted back into the woman.

The Instruction puts it this way:

> Thus moral conscience does not necessarily proscribe the use of certain artificial means destined solely either to the facilitating of the natural act or to ensuring that the natural act normally performed achieves its proper end. If the technical means facilitates the conjugal act or helps it to reach its natural objectives, it can be morally acceptable. If, on the other hand, the procedure were to replace the conjugal act, it is morally illicit.[16]

### Dignitas Personae[17]

The purpose of this document, released on September 8, 2008, was to bring the *Donum Vitae* up-to-date. Questions brought to the fore by advancing technology need to be answered, so the *Dignitas Personae* addresses research on human embryos and other areas of "experimental medicine." Society is reminded through this document "that the ethical value of biomedical science is gauged in reference to both the *unconditional respect owed to every human being* at every moment of his or her existence, and the *defense of the specific character of the personal act which transmits life*" (page 6, emphasis original).

Regarding the treatment of infertility, three fundamental goods must be respected. These are

(a) the right to life and to physical integrity of every human being from conception to natural death;

(b) the unity of marriage, which means reciprocal respect for the right within marriage to become a father or mother only together with the other spouse;

(c) the specifically human values of sexuality that require "that the procreation of a human person be brought about as the fruit of the conjugal act specific to the love between spouses" (page 7).

Therefore, fertilization in the laboratory is excluded, as is any substitution for the conjugal act. Treatments aimed at restoring natural function are allowed. Such treatments would include hormonal manipulation, and surgery to unblock fallopian tubes or correct endometriosis. Likewise, adoption is encouraged, but not embryo adoption, as noted later.

In consideration of IVF, the document decries the destruction of human embryos, whether intentional (as in preimplantation diagnosis) or unintentional (as in freezing and thawing, or multiple embryo transfers). It finds, "All techniques of *in vitro* fertilization proceed as if the human embryo were simply a mass of cells to be used, selected and discarded" (page 8). Specifically, intracytoplasmic sperm injection (ICSI) is deemed inappropriate, as is the cryopreservation (freezing) of embryos. As to those embryos currently frozen, the Church finds this a *"situation of injustice which in fact cannot be resolved"* (page 11, italics original). The cryopreservation of eggs, or oocytes, to be later used for "artificial procreation" is termed "morally unacceptable." Selective reduction of embryos or fetuses in the womb is called "intentional selective abortion" (page 12).

### Evaluation of Official Catholic Teaching

These very public publications of official Catholic teaching on procreation have generated a wide variety of reactions, from unqualified affirmation to total rejection. In our view, there is much in the official

## THE CATHOLIC CHURCH AND FROZEN EMBRYOS

Over 400,000 human embryos exist today in the U.S., stored away in containers of liquid nitrogen. The Catholic Church has spoken out against creating these embryos, foreseeing that the fate of the embryos would pose a serious dilemma. Brian Scarnecchia, the president of the International Solidarity and Human Rights Institute and a professor of law at Ave Maria Law School, gave a lecture addressing the issue at Pontifical Council for Justice and Peace. Traditionally, the Catholic Church has condemned surrogacy and in vitro fertilization, but now the Church must ask what is appropriate to do with the existence of frozen embryos. In 2008 the Congregation for the Doctrine of Faith issued *Dignitas Personae*. Paragraph 19 of *Dignitas Personae* stated that heterologous embryo transfer, the transferring of an embryo to a woman other than the mother of the embryo, was not permissible since it requires acts that are similar to in vitro fertilization and surrogacy. At the Pontifical Council, Scarnecchia argued that homologous in vitro fertilization is appropriate. For instance, it is appropriate for a mother who had in vitro fertilization and repented to take her frozen embryo back into her womb because the child has a right to gestational parenthood beneath his or her mother's heart.

Source: Andrea Kirk Assaf, "The Absurd Fate of Frozen Embryos," *Global Zenit News*, Feb. 25, 2010, Catholic.net.

Catholic teaching on procreation that is consistent with Scripture and that reflects the order of creation that was established in Genesis 1–2.

We would affirm that both sex and procreation belong to marriage and are restricted to the sphere of marriage. We further affirm that human life should be protected from conception forward and that any reproductive technology that involves the deliberate destruction of embryos is morally problematic.

Where we differ from the teaching of the Catholic Church is in its rigid insistence that procreation always come out of marital sexual relations. While we hold to procreation within the sphere of marriage, we do not insist that all procreative attempts originate with normal sexual relations. Thus we would suggest that it is possible to use IUI, IVF, GIFT, and ICSI without violating biblical teaching.

### Can the Two Aspects of Sex Be Separated?

To sharpen the point made above, we differ from the Catholic insistence that the unitive and procreative aspects of sex always go together every time a couple has sexual relations. The Vatican Instruction teaches that every act of sexual relations must be open to procreation, thus ruling out contraception and sterilization.

We would argue that the general connection between marriage and procreation must be maintained, but not every sexual encounter between husband and wife must encompass the unitive and procreative aspects of sex.

Catholic moral theologian Richard A. McCormick accepted the general link between marriage and procreation, but denied that both the unitive and procreative aspects must be present every time a couple has sexual relations. He stated, "it is sufficient that the *spheres* be held together, so that there is no procreation apart from marriage, and no full sexual intimacy apart from a context of responsibility for procreation."[18]

The Scripture affirms the essential goodness of both the unitive and procreative aspects of sex, but there does not appear to be any biblical demand that the two aspects always be linked. As we pointed out in chapter 2, the creation account establishes that the spheres of marriage and procreation be connected, but does not require that every time a couple has sexual relations, they be open to procreation.

The Scripture affirms that sex has a variety of purposes, all of which are ordained only within the confines of marriage. First, Scripture clearly teaches that sex is one of the means by which a couple experiences the physical oneness and spiritual unity that is a part of the mystery of marriage (Gen. 2:24; Eph. 5:29–33). Second, one of the ends of sexual activity in marriage is procreation; in fact, procreation is unique to sex as an end. Third, sex is designed for pleasure and is one of the ways a couple enjoys each other. Scripture views sex as good within marriage if it is an expression of a couple's love for each other. Within this context, any of the purposes for sex are good in and of themselves. In fact, sexual pleasure between married persons is good even if pleasure is the only mutual objective for any particular sexual act.

## Sex for Pleasure

The Song of Solomon bears eloquent testimony to the high place Scripture gives to sexual pleasure. The royal couple in the Song revel in each other's love, exhibiting a depth of passion that most couples would like to reproduce in their own marriage. The imagery of sex as a meal of choice foods (Song 4:13–5:1) indicates that pleasure was the objective of the couple on their wedding night. The way in which they describe each other's bodies in exquisite figures of speech (Song 4:1–7; 6:4–9; 7:1–8) makes it clear that pleasure is the purpose for the sex recorded in the book. Interestingly, in the entire book, there is not one mention of children or procreation. If the unitive and procreative purposes of sex must always go together, this is a most unusual omission. It seems to point to pleasure as an inherent and self-sufficient purpose of sex. That is, marital sex can be for pleasure alone, apart from any procreative intention.

Similarly in 1 Corinthians 7, Paul speaks of marital sex as a source of physical release and enjoyment, since it is better to marry than to burn with passion (v. 9). Paul commands that husbands and wives come together for sex regularly so that they will not be tempted to look elsewhere for the pleasure of sex (1 Cor. 7:2, 5; this seems to be the meaning of the phrase in verse 2, "since there is so much immorality"). They are commanded not to deprive each other, presumably of the pleasure of sex (and perhaps also the source of physical release), except by mutual consent for temporary periods of prayer and contemplation (v. 5). Husbands and wives are enjoined to fulfill their conjugal duties to each other (vv. 3–4) and nowhere in this passage does it mention children. Rather, in this passage the purpose of giving pleasure to one's spouse appears to be the sole and sufficient reason for sexual relations.

Of course, this does not remove the procreative aspect of sex since it is still a unique end of marital sexual relations. But the Scripture does not suggest that a procreative intention or openness to procreation must always be present every time a couple has marital sex. As we mentioned in chapter 2, we should be careful about reading too much into the descriptive fact that sex was required for procreation in biblical times. Of course there was a natural continuity between

## CATHOLICS DIVIDED ON EMBRYO ADOPTION

Roman Catholics are divided on the option of embryo adoption and the Catholic Church has not issued any authoritative statement on the practice as yet. Some Catholic theologians are encouraging infertile couples to adopt leftover embryos, as a rescue of embryonic persons that would otherwise be discarded or donated to research, which would result in their destruction. Other Catholic scholars are not so sure, suggesting that it violates the official Church teaching that procreation should occur as a result of normal sexual relations and that it allows for a cavalier attitude toward the creation of embryos in IVF procedures. They argue that embryo adoption makes couples complicit in IVF, which the Catholic Church opposes.

Source: Alan Cooperman, "Catholics Split on Embryo Issue," *Washington Post,* May 31, 2005, washingtonpost.com.

marital sex and procreation, since there were no other options for procreation outside of sexual relations. We suggest that procreation belongs to the general sphere of marriage, not necessarily to specific acts of marital sexual activity.

### Understanding the Position

Scripture does not demand a rigid link between the unitive and pro-creative purposes of sex. That being the case, then some birth control (separating out procreation) and some reproductive interventions (separating out the oneness and pleasure purposes) would seem to be morally legitimate.

Thus, if it is biblically allowed to separate the purposes for sex, and to separate the pleasure aspect from the procreative by using birth control, then it must be legitimate to separate procreation from sex by using some reproductive technologies.

We would suggest that the need for this connection between the two aspects of sex reaches an extreme in the Vatican view; this is echoed by some Catholic moral theologians. The Vatican Instruction affirms that sex does not lose its value, presumably in both its aspects, even when the couple is permanently infertile.[19] But it seems strange to assert that the sex act has procreative *as well as* unitive meaning even when the couple has no biological prospect of conceiving a child due to infertility or menopause.[20] In fact, menopause seems to be a natural, divinely ordained means by which the unitive and procre-ative aspects of sex are permanently separated. It makes little sense to affirm an openness to procreation after menopause.

In like manner, we would hold that some reproductive technolo-gies are acceptable even if they separate the unitive and procreative aspects of sex.

### Medical Intervention: Yes or No?

Another criticism of official Catholic teaching on procreation is that the prohibition of medical technology to alleviate infertility is arbitrary and overly restrictive, particularly in light of the Church's endorsement of medical technology in general. In other words, using medical technology to help couples alleviate infertility is generally as appropriate as using medical technology to treat other medical conditions.

The Instruction sanctions scientific research and technology as an expression of human beings' God-ordained dominion over the earth (Gen. 1:28). Science and technology cannot proceed apart from conscience and morality, however. There are considerations besides technological efficiency and progress that may place limits on the uses of such innovations. In view of this general support for technology as a legitimate exercise of human beings' dominion over creation, Catholic critics have found it odd and arbitrary that virtually no technology is allowed in the area of procreation. Since human beings are not only allowed, but entrusted, with extensive dominion over most other areas of life, it seems inconsistent to deny human beings the same dominion over sex and procreation.

Catholic teaching routinely allows for medical technology to intervene in order to restore malfunctioning organs and systems to their proper natural function. Many Catholic thinkers have difficulty understanding how reproductive technologies—which they view as essentially medical technologies—can be consistently excluded from legitimate medical treatment. Not only does medicine intervene; at times, it substitutes for a failing bodily function. For example, dialysis substitutes for diseased kidneys, ventilators substitute for diseased lungs, and pacemakers substitute for critical heart functions. In the same way, some reproductive technologies substitute for diseased fertility functions.[21]

Critics of the Church's position go even further and argue that the technological developments that enable human beings to more effectively exercise dominion over the creation reflect a part of our creative makeup that comes from our Creator. Professor Sidney Callahan suggests that "the mastery of nature through technological problem solving is also completely natural to our rational species; indeed, it is the glory of *homo sapiens*."[22]

### Common Grace

From a primarily Protestant perspective, this criticism is stated in terms of the notion of general revelation. As is true with new technology that serves the good of mankind, reproductive technologies are a part of God's general revelation that is universally available. As a part of creation and the mandate given to mankind to exercise dominion over the earth (Gen. 1:26), God gave mankind the ability to discover and apply all kinds of technological innovations.

It does not follow, however, that mankind has the responsibility to use every bit of technology that has been developed. But for the most part, technological innovations that clearly improve the lot of mankind are considered a part of God's common grace, or His general blessings on creation, as differentiated from His blessings that are restricted to those who know Christ personally.

This is even more so the case when the technology in question is being used to reverse an effect of the Fall. The use of medicine to alleviate infertility, a clear effect of the Fall, is parallel to the use of medicine to alleviate other physical effects of the Fall, namely, disease. It would appear that many of the reproductive technologies in question would fit under the heading of general revelation and common grace, and whether or not they should be used depends on whether or not such a use violates a biblical principle or text.

### Why Parents Want Children

Many commentators have pointed out that the strong desire of couples to have a child to whom they are genetically related is a nearly universal inclination. Though there may be some cultures in which this is not the case, for the majority of the human species there is a strong tendency not only to procreate but to pass on one's genetic material to the next generation. This is one reason infertile couples often oppose third party genetic contributors, and view adoption as a last resort.

Given the emphasis in Catholic teaching on the natural process of procreation, critics have wondered why the natural tendency to have a

---

**DISSENT FROM OFFICIAL CATHOLIC TEACHING**

Catholic theologian Charles Curran is among many voices in Catholic tradition that takes a different view of sexual and reproductive ethics. Curran argues that official church teaching is guilty of the error of biologism, or giving too high a priority to biological functions (or absolutizing the physical), at the expense of the goods of the human person and of the marriage. He suggests that at times, for the good of the marriage, it is acceptable to interfere with "the physical structure of the act (of sex)." On analogy with killing, the church does accept that sometimes the physical act of killing is acceptable, when other goods are served, such as self-defense. But when it comes to sexual relations, the act of sex has an intrinsic structure that cannot be violated. That, insists Curran, is inconsistent. Curran further argues that it is proper and necessary for church teaching to adapt, and he cites other examples, such as its views on religious liberty, that have evolved over the decades.

Source: Charles E. Curran, "Roman Catholic Sexual Ethics: A Dissenting View," *Christian Century* (December 16, 1987): 1139–42, http://www.religion-online.org/showarticle.asp?title=113.

---

genetically related child has been omitted from consideration. It would seem to be an integral part of the human procreative constitution. Further, it would seem that reproductive technologies, which can help fulfill that longing, should be considered morally appropriate.

Of course, this does not legitimate all measures to have a child. When medical technology can help fulfill this legitimate desire, however, it is curious that the Vatican, working from a natural law framework, has not included what seems to be a significant part of the human makeup. The Vatican might respond that, of course, the procreative intention is a significant part of human nature. But there are limits on how human beings can fulfill their normal human inclinations. For example, it would not be right to steal to fulfill the natural inclination to eat. In the same way, it is not morally legitimate to violate the inherent structure of sex in marriage to achieve a normal human longing.

### *Restoring a Natural Function*

But surely this is what medical technology is designed to do, to fulfill our innate human inclination for individual self-preservation by combating disease, one of the many effects of the entrance of sin into the world. And if it is true that the Vatican position reflects an overly narrow view of the relationship between sex and procreation and an arbitrary exclusion of infertility techniques from the realm of human technological dominion over the creation, then it would appear legitimate to use reproductive technologies to help fulfill the innate procreative constitution of human beings.

Reproductive technologies would be an extension of sex in marriage. Medical technology would provide that which the body can no longer do for itself, thereby restoring a natural function in order to fulfill a natural inclination. Infertility becomes a treatable obstacle.

## A Summary of Catholic Teaching

Official Catholic teaching has issued a negative moral judgment on most reproductive technologies. The insistence that the unitive and procreative aspects of sex must be inseparably linked is still the foundation for contemporary official Catholic teaching. Thus any technology that replaces normal sex is *not* morally legitimate.

Technologies that assist normal intercourse *are* morally acceptable within this framework. As a result, intrauterine insemination, in vitro fertilization, and surrogate motherhood have all been rejected. Couples like Maria and Alex need to be apprised of the Church's position, but not simply to be informed. They need an ongoing discussion, for many questions will arise. It seems reasonable that they would also understand the criticisms of the Church's position, and give careful thought and prayer to their decisions.

Such couples will hear that critics, from both inside and outside the Catholic Church, have argued that the official Church teaching in this area takes too narrow a view of sex and procreation and that the unitive and procreative aspects of sex in marriage can be legitimately separated. They may be surprised that the Church, which accepts medical technology in general, prohibits the use of reproductive technology. They will have to wrestle with the question of whether reproductive technologies necessarily separate the goods of marriage or, in fact, even promote some of them. And they will hear that the Church is underemphasizing the natural human inclination for a genetically related child.

## Our Response

Neither author of this book speaks from a Catholic position, although both respect the Catholic Church for her strong defense of life on many fronts. Both authors posit that medical technology as a whole is a gift, yet it is a gift to be used wisely and with due consideration. Medical technology is a part of God's general revelation to human beings, part of His equipment for human creativity, graciously given to the human race to enable us to exercise appropriate dominion over the creation. More specifically, since dominion in general clearly includes dominion over the human body, medical technology is one of God's greatest gifts to the human race, enabling human beings to overcome one of the principal effects of the entrance of sin into the world, disease. Infertility, though not a disease, is undoubtedly an effect of the fall of mankind into sin, and medical technology to reverse it is generally morally appropriate, within certain parameters.

Yet medical technology is also a gift over which we need to exercise appropriate dominion. Simply because it exists does not mean that all components of it are to be embraced. Proper biblical parameters of reproductive technologies include the use of the genetic materials of husband and wife. Such morally appropriate technologies include artificial insemination by husband, GIFT and ZIFT (zygote intrafallopian transfer),[23] as well as in vitro fertilization, within certain constraints.

To be sure, the Scripture looks skeptically at third party contributors. The Christian couple trying to conceive a child and be faithful to

Scripture at the same time needs to be very careful as they consider their options. The use of third party genetic contributors, as in egg or sperm donation, should be avoided. Likewise, surrogacy, with rare exception (see chapter 7), is not a recommendation of these authors. While there generally seems to be no compelling reason to prohibit infertile couples from using reproductive technologies, there are specific and excellent reasons for being very cautious.

The Catholic Church benefits us all by her careful consideration of these issues, even if we don't always agree with all the particulars of her stance.

*The moral status of embryos is not fundamentally a scientific question, but a philosophical one.*

# CHAPTER FOUR

# The Moral Status of Fetuses and Embryos

One of the fundamental philosophical issues underlying the discussion of reproductive ethics is the moral status and corresponding rights of fetuses and embryos. That is, who counts as a human person, and, more specifically, when does human personhood begin and end?

It will be argued that embryos and fetuses (hereafter referred to synonymously) are fully and equally human beings, and consequently, human persons.

How one views the unborn will, of course, greatly influence one's view of abortion. But it will also give some parameters for use of some new reproductive technologies. For example, if personhood begins at the point of conception, then embryos fertilized in vitro and kept in storage for further use are human beings.

Use of them for experimental reasons—or discarding them if they are not necessary—is morally problematic. In addition, if prenatal genetic testing reveals some genetic anomalies in the fetus, then the decision to end the pregnancy on that basis is very problematic, since it is a human being whose life is being taken. It is critical to properly understand the nature of the fetus/embryo in order to avoid moral difficulties in the use of the various reproductive technologies.

## The Nature of the Unborn in the Bible

Although the Bible never specifically states that the fetus (or embryo) is a person, it is misleading to suggest that the Bible has nothing to say on the subject.

The Bible does clearly prohibit the taking of innocent life in the sixth commandment, "You shall not murder" (Ex. 20:13). The biblical case is made by its equation of the unborn child in the womb with a child or adult out of the womb. In order to demonstrate that the unborn are persons, it is not sufficient to show that God is deeply involved in fashioning the unborn in the womb, and thus deeply cares about them.

Given His role as Creator of the entire universe, the same thing could be said of the animals. God is involved in the creation of animals and cares deeply for them as well. But from that alone, it does not follow that animals have the same status as persons, since God also gave mankind dominion over the animal kingdom.[1]

To support biblically the personhood of the fetus/embryo, one must show that God attributes the same characteristics of a person who has already been born to the pre-born one still in the womb. That is, the Bible must use person language in referring to the unborn. The passages that are cited below are not an exhaustive list of texts that could refer to the unborn, but represent the clearest passages that attribute the aspects of personhood to the unborn.

## Conceived and Birthed

In the account of the first birth, when Eve gave birth to her son Cain, this person language is used to describe Cain. In Genesis 4:1 (NASB), the text states that Adam "had relations with his wife Eve, and she conceived and gave birth to Cain, and she said, 'I have gotten a man-child with the help of the Lord.'" Here Cain's life is viewed as a continuity, and his history extends back to his conception. Eve speaks of Cain with no sense of discontinuity between his conception, birth, and post-natal life. The person who was conceived was considered the same person who was born.

This continuity between conception and birth is clearer in Job 3:3 (NASB), which states, "Let the day perish on which I was to be born, and the night which said, 'A boy is conceived.'" This passage employs what is called in Old Testament poetry a synonymous parallelism, in which the second line of poetry restates the first one, essentially saying the same thing in different language. The use of this type of parallelism enables one to say that the child who was born and the child who was conceived are considered the same person.

In fact, the terms "born" and "conceived" are used interchangeably in the passage, suggesting that a person is in view at both conception

### EMBRYOS FOR SALE

A Texas infertility clinic/adoption agency offered tailor-made embryos for sale to prospective parents. The Abraham Center of Life, based in San Antonio, announced that they were the first donor created human embryo bank in 2006 [only to be out of business by 2007]. The original idea of the bank was to allow couples to bring sperm and egg donors together to create embryos, which are then sold to the prospective parents. They can see photos of the donors at various stages of their lives.

Sources: Ronald Bailey, "Embryos for Sale: Is the New Service Ethical?," *Reason*, August 18, 2006.

and birth. What was there at birth was considered equivalent to what was there at conception. This is strengthened by the use of the term "boy" in the second half of the verse—not a thing or a piece of tissue that is a part of the woman's body that was conceived but a person.

This term for "boy" (Hebrew *geber*) is also used in other parts of the Old Testament to refer to a man and a husband (Ex. 10:11; Deut. 22:5); thus a person, in the same sense that an adult man of marriageable age is a person, was conceived on the night of Job's conception.

## God Knows the Unborn

Other passages describe God knowing the unborn in the same way He knows a child or an adult. For example, in Jeremiah 1:5, God states, "Before I formed you in the womb I knew you, before you were born I set you apart; I appointed you as a prophet to the nations." Here it seems clear that God had intimate knowledge of and a relationship with Jeremiah in the same way He did when Jeremiah was an adult and engaged in his prophetic ministry. He was already called to be a prophet when still in the womb.

A similar text occurs in Isaiah 49:1, which states, "Before I was born the Lord called me [literally, 'from the womb the Lord called me']; from my birth he has made mention of my name." Here the person in question was both called and named prior to birth, indicative of a personal interest that parallels the interest God takes in adults. It may be that this verse refers to preexistence before even the womb, since the person in view is the Suffering Servant, Jesus Christ.

A further indication that the unborn are objects of God's knowledge occurs in Psalm 139:13–16, in which it is clear that God is intimately involved in forming the unborn child and cultivating an intimate knowledge of that child. From a Christian worldview, this should be sufficient to discourage taking the life of the unborn since it interrupts the sovereign work of God in the womb.

However, the psalm further teaches a continuity of personal identity from the earliest points of pregnancy forward. The psalmist who is intimately known by God in the first few verses (see vv. 1–4) is the same person who was described as intricately formed in the womb by God later in the psalm. And he is the same person who, at the end of the psalm, requests God to search him and know his heart (v. 23).

One may object to the use of these texts by suggesting that all of these only refer to God's foreknowledge of a person prior to birth. However in most of these passages such as Genesis 4:1 and Job 3:3, it is clear that the person who eventually grows into an adult is the same person who is in view in the womb.

A second objection that is sometimes raised is that texts such as Psalm 139:13–16 only speak of a person being *formed* in the womb, not that the person in the womb is indeed already a person. However, one must make a distinction between a person who is developing in the womb and some other entity that is somehow maturing into a person. These texts indicate that in the womb from point of conception there is a person maturing; it is not some other being that will become a person at some point in the gestational process.

Two other passages attribute characteristics of personhood to the unborn and affirm the continuity of personal identity from the womb through adulthood. Psalm 51:5 states, "Surely I was sinful at birth, sinful from the time my mother conceived me." David here is confessing not only his specific sins of adultery with Bathsheba and the arranged murder of her husband, Uriah the Hittite (see 2 Sam. 11–12), but also his innate inclination to sin. This is a characteristic shared by all persons, and David's claim is that he possessed it from the point of conception. In addition, David is using a synonymous parallelism similar to its use in Job 3:3, and he appears to treat birth and conception as practically interchangeable terms. Finally in the New Testament, in Luke 1:41–44, the term "baby" is applied to a child still in the womb. The same term (*brephos*) is used to describe the newborn Jesus in Luke 2:16.

## Mary's and Elizabeth's Babies

Perhaps a more explicit reference to the significance of the birth of the baby (*brephos*) Jesus comes from the visitation of Mary to Elizabeth in the early days of her pregnancy.[2] Mary visits Elizabeth (Luke 1:39–56) only a few days after she has found out that she is pregnant with Jesus. The account of the angel's announcement (vv. 26–38) indicates that Mary left in haste to visit Elizabeth and share this news with her.

Allowing for travel time of roughly one week, when she arrives at Elizabeth's home, Mary is in the very earliest stages of her pregnancy, with a fetus—technically, embryo—that is less than two weeks gestational age. (This is actually not long in the process of embryonic development after which stem cells are harvested from embryos, and that embryos are frozen if they are intended to be stored for later use.)

### EMBRYOS DESTROYED FOR MINOR DISORDERS

New fertility regulations set by the British Human Fertilization and Embryology Authority (HFEA) allow doctors to destroy embryos that are affected by a list of certain genetic conditions, some which are not life-threatening or which may only be carried but never even developed in the baby. The list has 116 genetic conditions. Several of the conditions may not strike until late in life, such as cancer or blindness, and other conditions are not life-threatening and can be treated easily with medicine. Criteria used to choose which genetic conditions were on the list include: the general age of onset of the disease, the degree of impairment caused by the disease, and the medical treatment available for the condition. Embryos are screened for genetic conditions by the removal of cells from an embryo eight days after fertilization. If the embryo has one or more genetic defects then they are discarded, and healthy embryos are kept for implantation. Researchers admit that the use of selection for non-life-threatening defects is very controversial and can lead to a society where minor defects are deemed unacceptable and "abnormal."

Source: Lois Rogers, "Embryos Destroyed for 'Minor' Disorders," *Times Online*, Jan. 24, 2010, timesonline.co.uk.

Upon arrival at Elizabeth's home, Mary is immediately recognized as "the mother of my Lord" (v. 43). Even though she is carrying a very early stage fetus (in fact, at this point in the pregnancy, most expectant women do not even know they are pregnant) she is clearly recognized as a mother, and by implication, Jesus is recognized as her son, a baby. Further, John the Baptist leaps in Elizabeth's womb, perhaps signifying his recognition of the significance of Jesus' conception and in utero development.

### An Exceptional Passage?

The general tenor of Scripture supports the idea that the unborn are considered persons by God, described with many of the same characteristics that apply to children and adults. However, one passage in particular may indicate that the unborn is less than a full person. Exodus 21:22–25 (NASB) states, "If men struggle with each other and strike a woman with child so that she has a miscarriage, yet there is no further injury, he shall surely be fined as the woman's husband may demand of him, and he shall pay as the judges decide. But if there is any further injury, then you shall appoint as a penalty life for life, eye for eye, tooth for tooth, hand for hand, foot for foot, burn for burn, wound for wound, bruise for bruise."

Pro-choice advocates, for example, contend that since the penalty for causing the death of the fetus is only a fine but the penalty for causing the death of the mother merits the death penalty, the fetus must not be deserving of the same level of protection as an adult person. It must have a different status, something less than full personhood that merits life-for-life penalty if taken.

However, there is significant debate over the term translated "has a miscarriage." At best there is no scholarly consensus on the interpretation. The most likely translation is "she gives birth prematurely," implying that the birth is successful, only creating serious discomfort to the pregnant woman, but not killing her or her child.

The usual Hebrew word for miscarriage is the term *shakal*, which is not used here. Rather the term, *yasa'* is used. It is generally used in connection with live birth of one's child. The fact that the typical term for miscarriage is not used here and a term that has connotations to live birth is instead used suggests that the passage means a woman who gives birth prematurely.[3] This would make more sense of the different penalties accruing to the guilty party. And it may be that the following phrase in verse 23, "if there is serious injury," would apply to either the woman or to the child, so that if the woman actually did have a miscarriage, that would be punishable under the "life for life" scheme.

## Beyond the Womb

All of the biblical material just discussed makes the case for the personhood and right to life of the unborn child in the womb. However, an objection can be raised that what the Bible addresses is only applicable to the unborn *in the womb*. Since the biblical authors did not conceive of the notion of embryos existing outside the body, one can argue that they were not addressing the moral status of *extracorporeal* embryos, and thus claim that the Bible is silent on that issue. We would respond that the biblical teaching on the unborn does apply to embryos outside the body, and ultimately location does not make a morally significant difference. But to do that we need to use a different form of argument—philosophical instead of biblical. We will see that our philosophical view of embryos suggests a continuity of personal identity that begins at conception, with no morally relevant break in the process from conception to adulthood.

### *Moral Status: Science or Philosophy?*

It is important to see that the moral status of embryos is not fundamentally a scientific question, but a philosophical one. Science cannot conclusively determine philosophical matters by scientific observation alone. Science can tell us what kind of a biological entity an embryo is, whether it's alive, and even whether it's human (embryos that are the sources of stem cells are both alive and human, even when stored in the lab—if they were neither, scientists wouldn't be so interested in their stem cells).

But whether or not embryos are *persons* is not a biological question, but a philosophical one. It is not fundamentally a religious question, since one could arrive at the same conclusions apart from religious convictions, though theology does have something to say about the issue.

## Substance and Property-Thing

Developing a proper philosophical view of unborn human beings, whether fetuses or embryos, first requires drawing a distinction between substances and property-things. A substance is an individuated essence that exists as a deeply unified whole that is ontologically prior to and greater than its parts; that is, a substance is more than the aggregate or emergent sum of its parts and properties. Most importantly, a substance possesses a defining, internal principle within its essence that informs its ordered change and behavior.

By contrast, in a property-thing, there is no underlying bearer of properties existing ontologically prior to the whole, and no internal, defining essence that diffuses, informs, and unifies its parts and properties. It is merely a collection of parts, that, in turn, gives rise to a bundle of externally related properties that are determined by those parts.

To possess an internal nature, then, is possible only for substances, all of which belong to a natural kind and exist in a manner essentially unique to a particular class of beings. Their essential nature informs their being and affords the essential properties peculiar to their natural kind. All members of a given species exemplify the same essential nature.

So, while substances possess an internal nature, property-things, such as cars, do not. There is no internal, ordering principle to ground a car's unity, govern its lawlike change, or guide its movement toward an end or purpose. Instead, there are only modifications caused by external forces. Specifically, human minds designed and built the automobile by configuring its materials into a functional pattern. These materials had no inclination of themselves to be so structured, and are externally related in an artificial manner. The shape, location, and function of the materials could have been radically different, and each component could have been used for an entirely different purpose than constructing an automobile.

### Essence: According to Its Kind

By contrast, that which moves a puppy to maturity or an acorn to an oak tree is an internal, defining essence or nature. This nature directs the developmental process of the individual substance and establishes limits on the variations each substance may undergo and still exist. The acorn will not grow into a dog and the puppy will not become an oak tree. Consequently, a substance functions in light of what it is, and maintains its essence regardless of the degree to which its ultimate capacities are realized.

Thus, while physical form and the degree of functional expression may vary among members (individual substances) of a natural kind, such variance does not affect the essential nature of their being. For it is the underlying essence of a thing, not its contingent state of development at a given point, that constitutes what it is. We would not, for example, say that an oak sapling is of a different kind than an adult oak tree. As a substance grows, it does not develop into something different; rather, *it matures according to its kind.*

The actualization of its potentialities or capacities is both controlled by and a reflection of the substance's essential structure. The capacities for the acorn one day to develop a trunk, branches, and leaves are already embedded within the acorn, prior to their realization. This is true whether the acorn actually grows into a tree or not, since such development is dependent on conditions that are wholly independent of the acorn's essential nature. When such conditions are met, however, including the proper soil, environment, etc., the acorn will express its latent capacities in the fullest sense. The absence of such conditions is irrelevant to the essential nature of the acorn.

## Change and Identity

In addition, substances maintain their essential identity despite change, while property-things do not. An individual substance endures through change because it is more than the aggregate set of its parts, formed according to an external ordering principle. The parts or properties of a substance can change without altering the thing itself. This is true because it exists as a deeply unified whole that possesses these parts and properties.

A dog, for example, can lose a tooth or shed its fur, but remain the same dog throughout these processes of change; for the dog is not an aggregate sum of its parts, nor an emergent whole whose parts are prior to the whole. Instead, the whole is prior to the parts and these parts exist because of their internal relations to each other, grounded in the enduring essence of the dog.

By contrast, a property-thing is an ordered aggregate; that is, a whole that is constituted by its parts, and thus, it cannot sustain literal identity when it gains or loses parts. No single entity endures through change, but, instead, a successive series of ontologically distinct, though perhaps similar, entities that begin and cease to exist over time. Since property-things are identical to the sum of their bundled properties and ordered parts, a change in any property or part necessarily causes one "entity-stage" to end and another to begin. Thus, property-things have no enduring essences to ground their identity through change.

Our commonsense views of a human being strongly suggest that we correctly view a human person as a substance with a continuity of personal identity through time and change. Take, for example, our understanding of moral responsibility and criminal justice. Both assume a substance view of a person if they are to make any sense at all. The only way criminal justice can be meaningful is if the person being held responsible for a crime is actually the same person who committed it.

The same is true with holding someone morally responsible for things they have done. If someone commits a crime, and years later, if found out, is arrested and brought to trial, that person has undergone numerous changes to a variety of his or her accidental properties—in fact, every seven years, most of your cells recycle. Beyond that, they may have lost some important parts or seen other aspects change. Under a property-thing view of a person, that individual could plausibly argue that he is a different entity than the one who committed the crime some years ago. But such a claim would rightly be laughed out of court, precisely because the legal system presumes a continuity of personal identity through time and change—a substance view of a person—in order to hold someone accountable for crimes committed.

## Our View

We would argue that the Bible affirms a substance view of a human being. That is, human beings have an internal essence, a soul, which guides his/her physical maturity and provides a continuity of personal identity through time and change. We view many of the biblical texts cited above in defense of the personhood of the fetus to teach precisely this point—that human persons have a continuity of personal identity from the earliest points of pregnancy all the way through adulthood. For example, in Psalm 139, cited earlier, the Bible makes it clear that the psalmist David is the same person in the womb as he is as an adult. Similarly in Psalm 51, the passage affirms that David was the same person who was a sinner from conception as he was when he sinned with Bathsheba and against Uriah, her husband (2 Sam. 11–12).

In addition, the Bible clearly affirms that human beings have souls, the immaterial essence that provides the person with the ground of his or her identity—though we would also affirm that the norm for human persons is for souls to be embodied in a body-soul unity. This suggests a substance view of a human person is the view most consistent with the teaching of the Bible.

## When Does Personhood Begin?

One way to think about the moral status of the unborn, either fetuses or embryos, is with the following logical argument.

*Premise 1*: An adult human person is the end result of the continuous growth of the organism from conception.

*Premise 2*: From conception to adulthood, there is no break in this development, which is relevant to the ontological status of the person.

*Conclusion*: Therefore, one is a human person from the point of conception onward.[4]

Though few would deny premise 1, and the conclusion clearly follows from premises 1 and 2, the validity of premise 2 is the debatable part of this argument. To deny that the fetus/embryo is fully

### THE FATE OF NEW ZEALAND'S FROZEN EMBRYOS

According to the Human Assisted Reproduction Technology (Storage) Amendment Bill, frozen sperm, eggs, and embryos collected before 2004 must be destroyed in 2014 unless the Ethics Committee on Assisted Reproductive Technology says otherwise. The ethics committee is in the process of clarifying the rules for storing sperm, eggs, and embryos. Typically, sperm, eggs, and embryos can be kept for up to ten years, but there is an ongoing debate as to what date to consider the beginning of the ten years. The beginning of the ten years is generally considered either November 2004, when the act took effect, or from the point that the egg was first frozen and stored, whichever happened later. If the bill is passed then embryos will have to be destroyed after ten years, unless the Ethics Committee on Assisted Reproductive Technology grants permission to keep the eggs longer. The Advisory Committee on Assisted Reproductive Technology will set the guidelines for deciphering which eggs to grant, and which eggs not to grant, extensions.

Source: Audrey Young, "Fate of Frozen Embryos Rests with Ethics Board," *The New Zealand Herald*, March 31, 2010, nzherald.co.nz.

human from conception, one must point to an ontologically significant (substantial) modification that occurs between conception and birth. So far as we can tell, there is no good reason to believe that such a break occurs at any point in the process. In fact, we would argue that any distinction between a human being and a human person cannot be maintained, and such a distinction should be a red flag. Some disagree with this claim, however, and point to either "decisive moments" at which the fetus first acquires the status of human personhood or to functional criteria for humanness.

## Viability

The most common decisive moment, and the one currently endorsed by the Supreme Court, is *viability*, that is, the point at which the fetus is able to live on its own outside the womb. Currently, the average fetus is viable at roughly 24–26 weeks of gestation. Once this point is reached, some argue, the fetus acquires the status of personhood, by virtue of the fetus's ability to live on his/her own, though still dependent on medical technology—but not dependent on a uterine environment.

Viability as a determinant of personhood is unhelpful, because—if for no other reason—viability cannot be measured precisely. It varies from fetus to fetus, and medical technology is continually pushing viability back to earlier stages of pregnancy. Moreover, since viability continues to change, this raises questions about its reliability as an indicator of personhood. But proponents of viability argue it is possible, at least in principle, that medicine will reach a lower limit, say at twenty weeks gestation, and at this point, there may be no reasonable prospect of pushing it back any earlier. Given this scenario, viability will be a more stable concept, and thus it is argued that it is more reliable as a determinant of personhood.

But what does viability actually measure about a fetus? The concept of viability is a commentary, not on the essence of the fetus, but on the ability of medical technology to sustain life outside the womb. Viability relates only to the fetus's location and dependency, not to its essence or moral status. There is no inherent connection between the fetus's ability to survive outside the womb and its essential nature as a human being. Thus, while viability is a helpful measure of the progress in medical technology, it has no bearing on what kind of a thing the fetus is or is not.

## *Brain Development*

Perhaps the next most commonly proposed decisive moment is *brain development,* or the point at which the brain of the fetus begins to function, which is at roughly forty-five days of pregnancy. The appeal of this decisive moment is the parallel with the definition of death, which is the cessation of all brain activity. Since brain activity is what measures death—or the loss of personhood—some argue that it is reasonable to take the beginning of brain activity as an indication that personhood has begun.

This decisive moment, however, is unhelpful as well. The problem with the analogy to brain death is that the dead brain has no capacity to revive itself again. It is in an irreversible condition, but the fetus only temporarily lacks brain function. Its electroencephalogram (EEG) is only temporarily flat, whereas the dead person has a permanently flat EEG. In addition, the embryo from the point of conception has all the necessary capacities to develop full brain activity. Until around forty-five days gestation, those capacities are not yet realized but are latent in the embryo. However, that a capacity is not actualized has no bearing on the essence of the fetus, since that capacity is only temporarily latent, not irreversibly lost.

Thus, there are significant differences between the fetus for whom capacity for brain activity is latent in the first four to five weeks of pregnancy, and the dead person who lacks both the potentiality and the actuality for any brain activity whatsoever. Pointing to brain activity as the decisive moment for personhood, then, does not give a valid point at which personhood can be recognized.

## Sentience

A third suggested decisive moment is *sentience*, or the point at which the fetus is capable of experiencing sensations, particularly pain.[5] The appeal of this point for the determination of personhood is that if the fetus cannot feel pain, then there is less of a problem with abortion, and it disarms many of the pro-life arguments that abortion is cruel to the fetus.

As is the case with the other decisive moments, however, sentience has little inherent connection to the personhood of the fetus, since it confuses the experience of harm with the reality of harm. Simply because the fetus cannot feel pain or otherwise experience harm, it does not follow that it cannot be harmed. If I am paralyzed from the waist down and cannot feel pain in my legs, I am still harmed if someone amputates my leg.

In addition, to take sentience as the determinant of personhood, one would also have to admit that the reversibly comatose, the person in a persistent vegetative state (a person who has only the brain stem functioning), the momentarily unconscious, and even the sleeping person are not persons. One might object that these people once did function with sentience and that the loss of sentience is only temporary. But once that objection is made, the objector is admitting that something else beside sentience is determinant of personhood, and thus sentience as a decisive moment cannot be sustained.

## Quickening

Another suggested decisive moment is *quickening*, or the first time that the mother feels the fetus move inside her womb. Historically, this has been the first evidence of life to be detected clearly. This was obviously before the use of sophisticated medical technology such as ultrasound, which can see the fetus from the early stages of pregnancy.

Upon close examination, it becomes clear that quickening as a determinant of personhood is unacceptable because the essence of the fetus cannot be dependent on someone's awareness of it. This criterion confuses the nature of the fetus with what one can know about the fetus. In other words, this decisive moment confuses epistemology (knowledge/awareness of the fetus) with ontology (the nature or essence of the fetus).

## Appearance of Humanness

A similar confusion is involved in the use of *the appearance of humanness* of the fetus as the decisive moment for personhood. The appeal of this view is primarily emotional, in that as the fetus comes to resemble a baby, one begins to associate it with the kind of being that they would normally consider a full human being (e.g., a newborn). But what the fetus looks like has no inherent relationship to what it is, and from the point of conception, the fetus has all the capacities necessary to one day exemplify the physical characteristics of a normal adult human being. The appearance of the fetus, then, is an unhelpful criterion for human personhood.

## Birth

A few assert that *birth* is the decisive moment at which the fetus acquires personhood. Many pro-choice advocates who suggest that the law maintains neutrality on the moral status of the fetus actually default to this position. But we suggest that viewing birth as the critical decisive moment is deeply problematic. It seems intuitively obvious that there is no essential difference between the fetus on the day prior to its birth and on the day after its birth. The only difference between the pre-birth and post-birth fetus/newborn is her location, and the difference in the degree of dependence on the mother.

But as is the case with viability as the determinant of personhood, birth says nothing about what kind of thing the fetus is; it merely offers a commentary on her location. But just because I change venues, it does not follow that there is any essential change in my nature as a person. Likewise, just because the unborn human person changes his/her location, this does not change the fetus's essential nature as a fully human being.

## *Implantation*

A final suggested decisive moment is *implantation,* and proponents of this view offer at least three reasons in its defense. First, it is at implantation when the embryo establishes its presence in the womb by the "signals" or the hormones it produces. Second, since anywhere from 20–50 percent of the embryos spontaneously miscarry prior to implantation, some suggest that implantation is critical, not only to the development of the embryo, but to the essence of the embryo.

Proponents also suggest that if we claim that a full human person exists before implantation, then we are morally obligated to save every single embryo (something that very few people hold). Next, twinning, or the production of twins, normally occurs prior to implantation, and, according to some, this suggests that individual human personhood does not begin until after implantation.

Though placing personhood at implantation would have little effect on the abortion question (since induced abortions occur well after implantation), the ethical implications of this decisive moment are very significant. First, if correct, it would make any birth control methods that prevent implantation, such as the morning-after pill (Plan B), many forms of the birth control pill, and the "abortion pill," RU-486, morally allowable, since an embryo that has yet to implant is not considered a person. Further, leftover embryos that are kept in storage as part of in vitro fertilization could be discarded or experimented on without any moral problem, since those embryos do not possess personhood.

However, several things can be said against implantation as a decisive moment. First, just because the embryo establishes its presence by the hormonal signals it produces, it does not follow that personhood is established at this point. The essence of the fetus is independent of another's awareness of its existence, whether that awareness includes physical awareness, as in quickening, or chemical awareness, as in the production of specific hormones.

Second, just because up to 50 percent of conceived embryos

spontaneously miscarry, it does not follow that personhood comes at implantation, since the essential nature of the fetus is not dependent on the number of embryos that do or do not survive to implant. Moreover, even if the preimplantation embryo is a full human person, as we contend, we are not morally obligated to save each one since there is no moral obligation to interfere in the embryo's natural death. Not interfering to prevent a spontaneous miscarriage is not the same thing as killing an embryo any more than removing life support on a terminally ill patient and allowing him or her to die is not the same thing as actively killing such a patient.[6]

Third, just because twinning occurs prior to implantation, it does not follow that the original embryo was not a full human person before the split. In fact, it is equally possible that two persons existed prior to implantation, and only individualized after that point. Thus implantation fails to serve as an ontologically decisive moment for personhood.

## EMBRYO ADOPTION CUSTODY BATTLE

Two families are in a custody battle over embryos. A California family donated four frozen embryos to Jen McLaughlin. Both parties signed a contract that stated, the "pre-born children who are . . . entitled to the rights and protections accorded to all children legally and morally." Initially McLaughlin had two embryos implanted and gave birth to both children. She now wants to implant the remaining two embryos so her children can be raised with their siblings, but the California couple wants the remaining two embryos back so that they can give them to another couple. McLaughlin is now fighting to keep the children and the two non-implanted embryos together. The contract states that the donor couple has one year to seek and request the control of the remaining embryos. McLaughlin's attorney argues that the contract does not take into consideration that McLaughlin would be unable to embed the remaining embryos within the first year if the first two embryos implanted took.

Source: The original *St. Louis Post-Dispatch* article has been taken down; there is info at this site: culturecampaign.blogspot.com/2010/04/frozen-embryo-custody-lawsuit-to-set. html; more at contracostatimes.com/ci_15086092?source=most_viewed.

Proponents of implantation as the decisive moment insist that location does matter—that the womb is the only suitable place (as yet) for embryos to flourish and mature.[7] It is true that the various chemical environments in which IVF occurs and in which embryos are stored can only support embryonic development to a certain early stage. Until artificial wombs are available and workable, there is no substitute for a woman's uterus as a place of housing and nutrition for embryos and fetuses. However, it does not follow from this that implantation is the point at which an embryo obtains his/her moral status as a person.

Imagine that you were suddenly transported to the moon—an inhospitable place for human beings and entirely unsuitable for us to flourish. Of course, it would be morally wrong for someone to place you in such an incompatible place against your will. But just because you are in an environment that is unsuited for you to flourish, that is no necessary commentary on your moral status as a person.[8] Location is simply what it is—a different place, and nothing follows from a person's location concerning his or her moral and metaphysical standing.

Location does make a difference when it comes to the ability of the embryo to actualize its latent capacities, but as we've already argued, just because someone does not actualize particular capacities, it does not follow that they do not possess them. From the moment conception is complete, embryos possess all the capacities necessary to mature into a full-grown adult. The location in which it matures makes a difference only to the expression of those capacities—not to what kind of a thing it is ontologically.[9]

### Intuitive Attachment

But the notion that implantation is the decisive moment that counts for what makes someone a person has an intuitive appeal that is compelling at first glance. Take this hypothetical example. You are visiting the infertility clinic in which you have several embryos (created from the gametes of you and your spouse) in storage. Your two-year-old child is also with you at the clinic. Your child wanders off to a different part of the clinic about the time a fire breaks out in the area in which your embryos are being stored. It spreads so quickly that you do not have time to both find your child and gather your embryos and make it out alive. You must choose between your two-year-old and your embryos. Our intuitions tell us that this would not be a difficult choice—that you would grab your child and leave your embryos to perish in the fire. Critics of the view that embryos are persons maintain that this demonstrates that embryos and children cannot have similar moral status, since it is obvious that the parent values the child more than the embryos.[10]

The reason that our intuitions tell us to save our child is that we have strong emotional and relational attachments to our children. Those emotional factors are what drive our intuitions about who to save at the clinic. But emotional factors should not determine philosophical notions such as moral status and ontological value. For example, I would be much more distraught if my dog was run over in the street and killed than I would be if I read in the newspaper about the death of someone I do not know.

But one certainly could not conclude that my dog has more value ontologically than a person. It has more subjective value *to me*, but that subjective value cannot be the basis for a determination of its moral status and attendant rights to life. Similarly, in the clinic scenario, my two-year-old has more *subjective* value to me, based on the relationship I have with my child. But nothing follows in terms of the *objective* value of the embryos based on that emotional connection. At the least, one should hesitate before drawing conclusions of moral status and value based on emotional attachments and subjective factors.

## Being versus Functioning

Given the apparent inadequacies of the above decisive moments, philosophers such as Mary Ann Warren draw a more sophisticated distinction between a human being and a person, or between so-called genetic humanity and moral humanity, or between "biological life" and "biographical life."[11] Persons, or members of the moral human community, she claims, must meet one of five criteria:

1. Consciousness . . . and in particular the ability to feel pain
2. Reasoning, the developed capacity
3. Self-motivated activity
4. The capacity to communicate
5. The presence of self-concepts[12]

To this list, Joseph Fletcher adds (a) self-control; (b) a sense of the future and the past; (c) the ability to relate to others; and (d) curiosity.[13] The entire project of defining personhood in functional terms fails, since, as argued above, a thing is what it is, not what it does. Another way to put this is that *there is a difference between being a person and functioning as a person.*[14]

Simply because someone does not possess the capacity to exercise all the functions that persons normally do, it does not follow that he or she is not a person. An entity losing its function does not mean that the entity itself no longer exists, only that it cannot function, or perform all of its functions.

It is one thing if through neurological damage, I lose the ability to use my leg. It is quite another to insist that it is the same thing as losing my leg altogether. Even if I never had the use of my leg from birth and will never again have the use of it for the rest of my life, that is not the same thing as having it amputated. Just because some newborns cannot exercise many of the functions of personhood, and through deformity will never be able to exercise them, it does not follow that they do not possess the essence of personhood. Function is grounded in essence, and if function is absent, it is not necessarily a commentary on the essence of the unborn.

The weakness of attributing personhood based on function is that "to do" or "to function" has become synonymous with "to be." Yet as Catholic ethicist Richard Sparks puts it, "One's value is not wholly or even primarily ability-related. One's basic significance does not depend on the amount of functional abilities one has been endowed with nor on how well one exercises those talents."[15]

The inadequacies of functional definitions of personhood are clearly evident if we try to practice them consistently. Applying any of the above criteria, counterintuitive and ethically troubling results abound. Consider the person under general anesthesia. He is clearly not conscious, has no expressed capacity for reason, is incapable of self-motivated activity, cannot possibly communicate, has no concept of himself, and cannot remember the past or aspire for the future. According to the functionalist view expressed by Warren and Fletcher, he is not a full person—but this is absurd.

In response, it may be argued that the person is only temporarily unable to perform these functions. But this counterargument can only be made by appealing to something else besides the "critical functions" of a person outlined by Warren and Fletcher. Defending the personhood of the anesthetized human seems to require pointing to ultimate capacities that are embedded in his human nature. To argue that the person before anesthesia remains a person while under anesthesia, we must point to what that person is, irrespective of his functional capacities.

Finally, if essential personhood is determined by function, it follows that essential personhood is a degreed property. After all, some will realize more of their capacities to reason, feel pain, self-reflect, etc., than others. Moreover, it is undeniable that the first several years of normal life outside the womb include an increasing expression of human capacities.

Likewise, the last several years of life may include a decreasing expression of human capacities. Consequently, if the functionalist view is correct, the possession of personhood could be expressed by a bell curve, in which a human being moves toward full personhood in her first years of life, reaches full personhood at a given point, and then gradually loses her personhood until the end of her life. Presumably, the commensurate rights of persons would increase, stabilize, and decrease in the process.

## Ramifications of Functionality

Without appealing to something other than function, it is difficult to resist this counterintuitive conclusion. Indeed, intellectual honesty has driven some to embrace this end, and the slope is ever so slippery. Philosophers Helga Kuhse and Peter Singer comment on the ontological status of newborns:

> When we kill a newborn, there is no person whose life has begun. When I think of myself as the person I am now, I realize that I did not come into existence until sometime after my birth. . . . It is the beginning of the life of the person, rather than of the physical organism, that is crucial so far as the right to life is concerned.[16]

## THREE-PARENT EMBRYOS

Scientists have created a human embryo with DNA from three parents. The embryo was engineered to have nuclear DNA from two parents and mitochondrial DNA from a third parent. This type of technique is called germline genetic engineering, a process of altering DNA that passes on traits. Afraid that germline genetic engineering may lead to scientists creating designer babies or causing long-term health problems in the embryos, several countries, including France and Germany, have chosen to ban the practice. Nonetheless, much more research is needed before a three-parent embryo can be fully developed. The procedure was first used in mice and monkeys. While the engineered mice have grown normally, researchers have yet to discover whether the monkeys will mature normally since they are still young.

Source: Brandon Keim, "3-Parent Embryos Could Prevent Disease, but Raise Ethical Issues," *Wired Science*, April 14, 2010, Wired.com.

While we applaud their intellectual consistency in applying their notion of personhood evenly in ethical issues, their chilling consistency reveals the danger of defining human personhood in functional terms. Not only are the unborn—and newborns—less than persons, apparently all of us are subject to graded personhood and the commensurate rights therein.

To be a human person is to possess an essential human nature. The unborn are individual human substances, possessing an essentially human nature; therefore, they are human persons. Functional definitions of personhood are arbitrary, metaphysically inadequate, and ethically problematic. Essence precedes function—to possess an essential human nature is to be a human person, regardless of whether one's functional capacities are actualized or not.

## In Conclusion

The use of embryos in some reproductive technologies raises the question of the moral status of early stage embryos, particularly those that exist outside the womb (ex utero embryos). Some suggest that such microscopic entities that consist of a group of cells cannot possibly be a person. Others insist that size and location are irrelevant to a being's ontological and moral status, and that the continuity of personal identity that applies to fetuses extends to embryos too.

Our common views of a person assume a continuity of personal identity, which requires a substance view of a human being. Our social notions of moral responsibility and criminal justice are dependent on this view of personal identity. We assume that when we bring someone to trial for a crime that had been committed years prior, we are trying the same person who committed the crime, regardless of how that person has changed or how much time has elapsed.

Being a person, then, is a matter of one's *essence*, or nature, not the ability to perform certain functions. If being a person is determined by our ability to perform certain functions, such as having self-awareness, relationality, and others, then personhood ends up being a degreed property, something of which one can have more or less. But if personhood is an essential property, then it is an all-or-nothing property, with the result that one either is or is not a person. Only an essential view of a person avoids the problematic idea that being a person is a matter of degree. Once it is admitted that being a person is a matter of essence, then the continuity of personal identity follows. Once a continuity of identity is established, then there is no place along the continuum from conception to birth where there is a valid "decisive moment" at which an embryo/fetus becomes a person. As a result, *one is a person from conception forward*. The single cell embryo has all the information it needs to mature into a full-grown adult, needing only shelter and nutrients. If implantation does not make a morally relevant difference, as we maintain that it does not, then whether embryos are implanted in the womb or are stored in the lab is irrelevant to their moral and ontological status.

Both philosophical reason and the testimony of Scripture suggest that fetuses and embryos are persons from the point of conception, with all the attendant rights to life. In utilizing the various reproductive technologies, one should be aware that fetuses and embryos are not items that can be discarded if no longer wanted or necessary. Couples who plan on using technologies that involve fertilizing and storing embryos in the lab should plan accordingly to ensure that human life, even if only in embryonic form, not be taken lightly. Further, if prenatal testing is used, couples should be aware that fetuses, even if genetically defective, are nonetheless persons, whose right to life deserves protection. Couples should enter into the various reproductive technologies with the awareness that they are creating human persons in whatever process they use—human persons for whom they are responsible.

# PART II:

# Evaluating Procedures

---

Intrauterine Insemination
and Egg Donation

GIFT, ZIFT, and IVF

Surrogate Motherhood

Prenatal Genetic Testing

*If, what, and when to tell the child about his or her genetic origins are not easy issues to address.*

# CHAPTER FIVE

# Intrauterine Insemination and Egg Donation

When we met Alex and Maria earlier in chapter 3 (Catholic natural law and procreation), they were struggling with their infertility and asking questions about which of the assisted reproduction techniques might be an option for them. They initiated a series of meetings with their priest, and underwent further testing at Dr. Davis's office. It was in the midst of all this that they attended a community fund-raiser, and were surprised to be seated at the same table as Robin and Bruce.

The conversation turned to family matters, and Robin talked about how Charlie's birth had upended their lives in amazingly wonderful as well as challenging ways. She mentioned that, because of her age, she had undergone fertility treatment, which, in her case, included egg donation from a younger woman. Maria wondered about the woman offering her eggs: How did that work?

As Alex and Bruce walked to the dessert table, Alex remarked that they were facing infertility issues as well. Bruce had two comments for Alex. He stated that egg donation cost a lot of money, and that his sperm were great swimmers. He knew this because he had provided both.

Suddenly, Alex just wanted to go home.

After all the appropriate testing of Maria and Alex was completed, they were reassured to learn that both their reproductive systems seemed to function just fine. Dr. Davis could not pinpoint any specific reason why they had not become pregnant. While they were relieved about this, it seemed to leave them in unmarked territory. Should they just keep trying on their own, or add fertility drugs? Should they consider IVF or gamete donation?

Although the Catholic Church's position did not allow for either of these, Maria decided that she would investigate both of these options further, so she and Alex could make an informed choice when the time came to choose. What she found surprised her.

## The Nature of Embryos

The use of embryos in some reproductive technologies raises the question of the moral status of early stage embryos, particularly those that exist outside the womb (ex utero embryos). Some suggest that such microscopic entities consisting of only a handful of cells cannot possibly be a person. Others insist that size and location are irrelevant to a being's ontological and moral status, and that the continuity of personal identity that applies to fetuses extends to embryos too.

This viewpoint is specifically relevant to IVF, in which the common practice is to maximize the number of embryos available for implantation; this results in embryos being left over. If embryos are persons with moral status and the right to life, then that makes a significant difference in how a couple approaches IVF. In addition, this discussion of the moral status of fetuses, which the biblical texts more directly address, is relevant to technologies such as IUI (when used with IVF fertility drugs, thereby running the risk of major multiples of pregnancies), and IVF and the sometimes recommended practice of selective termination of pregnancies. We will elaborate further on these applications in the chapters that address the specific technologies.

## *An Overview of IUI*

In this chapter, you will be introduced to some of the most widely used, least expensive, and least technically complex techniques, as well as to the most expensive and least used techniques to assist a couple in having a child.

Intrauterine insemination (IUI), either by husband or by donor (DI), is a relatively inexpensive treatment to counter male infertility. The female equivalent, egg donation, is much more complicated and expensive.

Egg donation is used when a woman cannot produce eggs, or, for some genetic reason, the couple does not want to use the eggs she produces. This is not typically a treatment for blocked fallopian tubes. Through either DI or egg donation, the child born will have a genetic connection with only one parent. If another woman contributes the egg, then only the father will be related genetically to the child; conversely, if DI is used, only the mother will have a genetic link with the child.

Intrauterine insemination by donor may be a relatively simple and inexpensive intervention, but it raises complex moral issues. Egg donation also raises many ethical and moral issues and is both complicated and expensive besides.

To be clear, be aware that the use of the term "donation" for both eggs and sperm is a bit misleading, since the donor is paid for the "donation." In our view, this actually constitutes the sale of eggs and sperm. The law makes an exception to the general prohibition of selling body parts in the case of eggs and sperm, but to call them donations does not accurately describe the transaction taking place.

However, we will use the standard terminology—sperm and egg *donation*—in order to avoid confusion.

In chapters 2 and 3, which laid out the biblical and theological material related to procreation, we concluded that the ideal setting for reproduction was a heterosexual married couple. This appears to be the pattern that God set up at creation. We rejected natural law conclusions that would restrict most reproductive interventions as inconsistent with the notion of general revelation. Technology that bettered the lot of the human race and helped alleviate an effect of the fall of mankind into sin is generally acceptable within specific biblical parameters.[1] Most reproductive technology fits in this morally allowable category. Thus the Christian can cautiously use a number of reproductive technologies within biblical guidelines.

## The Third Party

We also concluded that though the Bible is skeptical about reproductive technologies that involve a third party (as a genetic or gestational contributor), it does not clearly and unequivocally prohibit them. Techniques that require a third party contributor, however, should give Christian couples much pause. Many instances of intrauterine insemination and all egg donations require this kind of third party contributor, and thus, the issue of morality arises. For many couples, the major moral impediment to using intrauterine insemination by donor is that it involves use of donor genetic material. Since that issue was addressed in chapter 2, we will not revisit those arguments here.

The intent in this chapter is to address other moral and pragmatic concerns raised by use of intrauterine insemination and egg donation that should be contemplated by any couple, Christian or not, who considers using these.

## Beginnings

Intrauterine insemination (IUI) has a long history in animal husbandry, and was first used in humans as IUIH (intrauterine insemination by

## UK WOMEN TAKING RISKS IN ONLINE SPERM BANKS

In 2005 Britain passed a law that removed the right for donors to be anonymous; as a consequence fewer men are willing to donate sperm, and the UK is experiencing a shortage of sperm donations. A national shortage of sperm donors in the UK is leading women to use fertility clinics online or travel abroad to find sperm donors. Infertility clinic specialists are worried because many online clinics do not screen donated sperm for diseases, such as HIV and hepatitis, whereas in Britain, fertility clinics are required to keep sperm for six months after and then test it for infection. The clinics online avoid regulations in Britain by claiming that the company merely act as "agents" who connect sperm recipients and donors, but do not deal directly with the sperm. The risk of traveling abroad to retrieve sperm donations can be risky since many countries have more relaxed laws on sperm donation. In response to the decline of donors the Human Fertility and Embryology Authority is considering reforming the law.

Source: Kate Devlin, "Donor Shortage 'Driving Women to Risky Online Sperm Banks,'" *The Telegraph*, Jan. 22, 2010, telegraph.co.uk.

husband) in the late 1700s by John Hunter, an English physician.[2] Then in 1909, a report of donor insemination was published: a young American wife's husband was sterile; they sought help at a medical school, and the problem was solved in a novel way. Unbeknownst to the woman, she was inseminated with the sperm of the "best looking" medical student in the professor's class, and became pregnant.[3] With such beginnings, it perhaps is no surprise that, due to widespread religious and social opposition, DI was not widely used until the 1960s.

### *Keeping Tabs*

How often intrauterine insemination is done today in the United States is remarkably unclear. The Congressional Office of Technology Assessment (OTA), which provided data to the U.S. Congress for twenty-three years, closed in 1995.[4] The OTA conducted a survey of intrauterine insemination in 1986–87. Approximately 172,000 women were inseminated during that time, with 65,000 births resulting. Thirty thousand of those births were from donor insemination.

Insemination that does not accompany IVF is not reported to the Centers for Disease Control and Prevention, and there is no entity that collects DI data now. Infertility clinics, obstetricians' offices, sperm banks, and do-it-yourself kits are sources for DI. It seems not unreasonable to estimate that since the 1960s, a million births in the United States have originated from intrauterine insemination by donor.[5]

Who donates sperm? Traditionally, it has been students, like the "best looking" one described above. Sperm banks in the United States typically advertise for young males, college age to late thirties, in good health, with no significant family medical history of inheritable diseases. The potential donors are of medium height or greater, heterosexual, and legally able to work in the United States.[6] Many donor clinics are willing to help provide the couple with a match for certain traits such as hair color and texture, eye color, ancestry, skin tone, height, and blood type. Donors may be "anonymous" or "open."[7] At least one sperm bank offers a "Doctorate Donor" category.[8]

## Guidelines for Sperm Donation

The American Society for Reproductive Medicine publishes guidelines for sperm donation;[9] the American Association of Tissue Banks and the Food and Drug Administration (FDA) regulate sperm banks. The guidelines are not laws, but the regulations have some teeth. Many sperm banks state online that they follow the regulations. There is one primary exception: in 2005, regulations came into effect (several years after they had been written) stating that sperm donors could not have had same-sex intercourse in the previous five years. There was some protest about this, and at least one sperm bank openly does not follow this regulation.[10]

Individuals who donate sperm are paid—usually $60–$100 per acceptable sample.[11] The range paid depends on certain sperm qualities.[12] Sperm banks often ask for two or more donations each week from approved donors, and many donate sperm regularly for months to years.

The payment has been welcomed by students, and some have continued to donate for years. One medical student began donating sperm two times per week in 1980, and continued that for fourteen years. By his estimation, he may have four hundred offspring. Now he is concerned about his genetic children perhaps dating one another, and has made his genome available on the Web through Harvard's Personal Genome Project.[13]

The qualifications for donating sperm have changed over the last decade or two. Potential donors are typically tested for several infections—HIV, Hepatitis B and Hepatitis C viruses, Chlamydia, and bacteria that cause syphilis and gonorrhea, all of which can be sexually transmitted. The medical history review, examination, and testing of the potential donor adds to the cost of DI. The costs of DI are based on the costs of paying the donor, testing of the donor and the sperm, storage of the sperm (if cryopreserved, or frozen), the clinic overhead, and the profit margin required. Even so, DI remains one of the least expensive of the reproductive technologies.

### Egg Donors

Egg donation is a different story. It is both more involved and more expensive than sperm donation. But that is not to say that there is no demand or market for donated eggs. With more women waiting longer to start families, it should not be surprising that the need for donor eggs would be increasing. In some cases, the women seeking donated eggs are past childbearing age; that is, they are postmenopausal and a donated egg is the only way for them to have a child. In 1990, there were reported in the United States just over five hundred egg donations.[14] By 2006, egg or embryo donations composed 12 percent of the ART cycles, or 16,976 cycles.[15] (See page 24 for "cycles.")

Who donates eggs? In some cases, it is a sister, other relative, or friend/acquaintance. In far more cases, it is a commercial arrangement, at least in the United States. Potential egg donors undergo not only health screening but psychological screening as well. The donation process itself requires oral and injected medications, which cause more than the usual one egg per month to mature and be released. Then a laparoscopic procedure that requires anesthesia is performed to retrieve the eggs. Usually five to twenty eggs are retrieved. The payment of $5,000–$50,000 per donation cycle is not dependent upon the number of eggs retrieved.[16] Although the American Society for Reproductive Medicine has issued guidelines for payment for egg donation, these are not necessarily followed.[17] Egg donors receive higher payments if they have had a successful pregnancy—either themselves or through a donated egg; have high SAT scores; are musically gifted or athletically accomplished; or have a variety of other characteristics, including desired physical features.

The physical toll for donating eggs is varied, but can be high. The risk of ovarian hyperstimulation syndrome, while low overall, is a serious one. Julia Derek who, as a beautiful young Swedish woman at an American university donated her eggs, tells her story in *Confessions of a Serial Egg Donor*. Despite her near-death experience in the process, she donated eggs twelve times—for the money. Her description on the back of her book is an important one: "Julia Derek is a writer who lives in New York City. Her eggs are no longer available to the public."[18]

The costs incurred by the recipient are dependent on the amount paid to the donor, fertility drugs to both the donor and the recipient (whose cycles must mesh for the process to take place), and the IVF process. The baseline price is usually $20,000, but varies widely.[19]

Egg donation is sometimes done in conjunction with IVF egg retrieval. The woman undergoing egg harvesting for IVF can designate some of the eggs to be donated, normally to a specific person. This kind of donation does not happen that often because women undergoing IVF are motivated to harvest and fertilize as many eggs as possible, in order to keep the costs down and the success rate up. Many clinics that offer egg donation services require that the woman who needs the eggs provide her own donor. So there is some anonymous egg donation, but its frequency is not anywhere near the incidence of anonymous sperm donation.

## Protection for Children

In limited ways, the law protects the children born from DI and egg donation. The Uniform Parentage Act states, "The donor of semen for use in intrauterine insemination of a married woman other than the

---

### RAFFLING DONATED EGGS

The Bridge Centre in London started a new service in March 2010 that allows women in the UK to utilize egg donation services in America. To kick off the start of the new service the IVF clinic raffled a donated human egg. The winner of the egg would have the egg implanted through IVF at the Genetics and IVF Institute (GIVF) in Fairfax, VA. Many were upset with the idea of both raffling eggs and using egg donors from the United States, where women are paid large sums of money for their eggs. The laws for egg donation differ in the US and the UK. In the UK eggs cannot be sold for profit (women often get paid around 250 pounds for a treatment), donors cannot be anonymous, and they can legally be contacted by the offspring at the age of eighteen. In response to the strict laws, there is a shortage of egg donors. The director of the Bridge Centre said that the new service was in response to the shortage of egg donations in the UK. The £13,000 procedure includes giving egg recipients the opportunity to acquire personal information of the egg donors, such as education, health, upbringing, race, and so on. The background information is meant to enable recipients to try and select eggs that will end up looking similar to them.

Sources: Ailsa Taylor, "UK Clinic Launches Overseas Egg Donation Service," BioNews, March 15, 2010, Bionews.org.uk.
"British Fertility Clinic Raffling Human Egg," Google.com, March 14, 2010.
Dr. Vivienne, Raper, "Exclusive: 'Rafflegate' Doctor Says Brits Travelling to US for IVF," BioNews, March 21, 2010, Bionews.org.uk.

donor's wife is treated in law as if he were not the natural father of a child conceived thereby."[20] The reason for this presumption, that the legal father of the child is the husband of the woman who gives birth to the child, is twofold. First, to protect the child from the stigma of illegitimacy, and then to ensure that the child is financially provided for. Normally when a man donates sperm, he signs a waiver of parental rights to any child conceived from use of his sperm. Thus, even if the donor should discover who used his sperm, which would be very difficult when the donation is anonymous, he would be prohibited from successfully claiming paternal rights to the child. Most states do not greatly regulate intrauterine insemination and egg donation except to provide for parental rights for the child.

### Moral Considerations and IUI

There is general agreement that intrauterine insemination with the husband's sperm (IUI) is morally allowed under most circumstances. The exceptions to this are the adherents of Roman Catholic natural law, who hold that any technology that replaces normal sex is not in keeping with the natural reproductive process that God instituted at creation. The official Catholic opposition to IUI is based on the fact that masturbation is needed to collect the sperm from the husband. In their view, that act constitutes replacement of sex, not just assistance.

However, some Catholic thinkers suggest that IUI can be used in conjunction with the normal sexual act so that it only assists and does not replace it. They advise a sheath style condom that seals after the initial expulsion of semen during sex, thereby collecting the sperm. The sperm would then be treated and the wife would be inseminated with it. This way of collecting sperm is not the typical manner in which infertility clinics do IUI, primarily because the initial ejaculate contains the most sperm.

For the Christian who accepts reproductive technology in general, there is no reason to hesitate to use IUI. It is true that the process does depersonalize procreation to some degree, but for most couples, that is a minor and acceptable price to pay for the technological assistance that helps them conceive a child.

## IUI with Fertility Drugs

One new way in which IUI is being used is in conjunction with the same drugs that are used in IVF to enable a woman to ovulate more than one egg during a particular cycle. She is given fertility drugs and, at the right time during the cycle, is inseminated with her husband's sperm. This increases the chances of achieving a pregnancy since in most cases, more eggs are released into the fallopian tubes.

The risk of this is similar to the risk in IVF, that there might be more than one pregnancy that would result. A couple who intends to employ this combination of reproductive assistance should be aware of the risk of a multiple pregnancy. Typically, selective termination, or abortion of one or more embryos or fetuses in the womb, will be offered. For the Christian couple, selective termination of one or more of the pregnancies, should they become pregnant with more children than they planned on or desire to rear, is not a morally appropriate option.[21]

## Complications and Egg Donation

There are both moral and pragmatic questions about DI and egg donation that must be considered by any couple contemplating use of these procedures. Couples who consider using DI and egg donation should become fully aware of the potential problems and moral issues involved. It has been widely assumed in medical circles that intrauterine insemination is relatively risk free, and that in most cases there are no medical complications.

Egg donation is more complex. In 2005, the European Parliament adopted a resolution calling for a ban on human egg trade, and for human egg donation to be more strictly regulated, because of the risks, including hyperstimulation, to the women involved.[22] In the United States, there is no long-term study of the risks involved. Further, the long-term effects of the medications used are unknown.[23]

Jennifer Lahl, of the Center for Bioethics and Culture Network (cbc-network.org), has collected stories of women whose lives have been adversely affected by egg donation. Several deaths have been recorded in the literature, usually stemming from ovarian hyperstimulation, when too many eggs have developed: the body retains much fluid, and multiple organs—lungs, kidneys, heart—are involved.

Another concern is the development of cancer. One infertility specialist in the UK reported the death of a woman who had been an egg donor. When she was thirty-two, she had donated six eggs to her

## NEED FOR FOLLOW-UP OF EGG DONOR RISKS

Over 100,000 young women in the United States have been egg donors, yet an extensive research of the emotional, psychological, and physical well-being of egg donors has yet to be had. Dr. Jennifer Schneider of Arizona Community Physicians helped conduct a research of egg donors' experiences, and the possible short- and long-term effects of egg donation. The survey included donors' medical complications, health problems, emotional state, and the amount of contact with the IVF clinics after the donation. The study revealed that a high percent of women had ovarian hyperstimulation syndrome, infertility, and menstrual problems. Also, 96 percent of women were never contacted by the IVF center for medical updates. Not only are women uninformed of the possible risks of egg donation, IVF clinics have yet to keep good medical records of egg donors. The best way to make research possible may be creating a national egg donor registry so that researchers can contact donors when needed. Dr. Schneider notes that fertility clinics focus solely on serving infertile women but clinics need to expand their responsibilities to taking care of egg donors and egg donor recipients. According to Schneider, an efficient fertility clinic should have long-term medical records of donors, fully inform women of possible risks, and help the needs of egg donor recipients.

Source: Jennifer Schneider, "Egg Donors Need Long-Term Follow-Up: Recommendations from a Retrospective Study of Oocyte Donors in the US," Progress Educational Trust, Jan. 19, 2009, IVF.net.

infertile younger sister. Several embryos were frozen, and a baby girl was born. When the infertility center tried to contact the donor a few years later about the disposition of the extra embryos, they learned she had died of widely metastatic colon cancer shortly before her thirty-ninth birthday.[24] Other risks of egg donation are bleeding and infection, based on the fact that a (minor) surgical procedure is done to "harvest the eggs."

In addition to these medical, physical, and pragmatic concerns about sperm or egg donation, there are also moral questions.

## *Is It Adultery?*

One of the most common preliminary questions about DI specifically is whether or not it constitutes adultery. Adultery is defined as a married person having sex with someone beside his or her spouse. DI does not involve sexual intercourse between the donor and the woman.

In the normal practice of DI, the consent of the husband is necessary prior to his wife being inseminated. Thus, even though the sperm of another person beside her husband is placed into her uterus, the husband's prior consent makes DI entirely unlike adultery, in which the husband usually does not know anything about his wife's affair and she does everything she can to keep it a secret.

DI is normally done openly (although the identity of the donor is usually not known). This is important, since what makes adultery a particularly egregious sin is that it involves such a deep betrayal of trust and a violation of the covenant of marriage.

Consent of the husband alone, however, does not exempt DI from the charge of adultery. Suppose two couples consent to have an "open marriage" in which they share sex with each other's spouse. It is done openly with nothing to hide. Even though there is technically no betrayal of trust, the practice still constitutes adultery because they were engaging in sexual relations with someone outside of the marriage partnership. Consent actually in this case is irrelevant in determining whether or not the people in this open marriage ha committed adultery. Neither a one flesh relationship nor a betrayal of trust occurs during normal DI. Thus it is hard to see how consensual DI could be a violation of the seventh commandment, which prohibits adultery (Ex. 20:14).

### Should Single Women Use DI?

DI makes it possible for single heterosexual women and lesbians to bear children. Many Christian women who strongly desire to have children and would undoubtedly make wonderful mothers cannot fulfill that dream because they have not yet met husbands. So they turn to DI or adoption as alternatives to have a family.

The law is beginning to look more favorably on single women adopting children and at present the law does not prevent any single woman from pursuing intrauterine insemination. However, some clinics will not perform the procedure on a woman unless she is married. Others require evidence to show that the child will be cared for adequately by the woman, and it is helpful if she can show that the child will have input from some male figure.

Even though the law allows single women to undergo DI, is it advisable for them to do so?

A single woman should be very careful before employing DI to help her start a family. The ideal of children being born into heterosexual marriages is intentional, to have both male and female input and role models for the child, both of which are necessary for healthy child development.

This is not to say that single parent families that result from divorce or death of a spouse are any less genuine families or that single parents do not frequently do a great job as parents. But there is a significant difference between single parenthood that comes about by unintended tragedy and that which comes about by intentional preplanning.

Single parenthood that results from divorce or death is a situation in which everyone attempts to make the best of a difficult situation.

The clear pattern in Scripture is that children are to be procreated into a stable family setting founded by a married heterosexual couple. Just because single parenthood is acceptable in the emergency scenarios of divorce and death does not mean that it is acceptable when those emergency conditions do not exist. This would seem to suggest that lesbians could not use DI to have a child and be consistent with Scripture. It would also suggest that single heterosexual women should not also use DI to fulfill their dreams of starting a family.

One may object by pointing out that this model of procreation is not black-and-white, and that even Scripture itself allowed some exceptions to this general rule, thereby perhaps opening the door for third party contributors. But in most cases of DI and egg donation contemplated to this point, that has involved a third party donor to a stable heterosexual couple. That is, the child will still be born into a stable heterosexual family according to God's original design. Even in the cases of surrogacy in the Old Testament, the infertile couple was a stable heterosexual couple who took full responsibility for rearing and supporting the child. Though the means used to procreate the child were deviations from God's original model, the setting into which the child was born was not.

So even when Scripture is not crystal clear about the means of procreation, it does seem clear about the setting into which children are to be born, consistent with what we know about the best interests of the child.

### The Tough Job of Single Parenting

Other pragmatic considerations that seem to advise single women against bearing children by DI are the rigors of rearing a child alone. Single parents undoubtedly have one of the most demanding responsibilities of any group in society, and a single woman should think long and hard before voluntarily taking it on.

For example, evidence is accumulating that shows the need for children to have present, involved fathers in their lives. A growing body of evidence indicates a connection between things like school dropout rates, delinquency and crime, and the lack of a father in the home.[25] Nearly 40 percent of children born in the United States in 2007 were born into single parent families.[26] Given the impact of a dad's absence in the life of a child, society should think very carefully before condoning the intentional creation of no-dad families.[27]

Ethicist Daniel Callahan of the Hastings Center correctly questions the wisdom of intentionally creating families without a father present through use of DI for single women.[28] Though most single mothers can make arrangements to have male influences for their children, it is usually only periodic at best and not equivalent to having a two-parent family in which the father is active in the child's life.

To be sure, there are situations in which that is not possible due to the father's abandoning his responsibilities or to a mother being widowed. Then the mother does the best she can with the resources she has and she should be commended for her efforts. Many had no idea that it would be so demanding when they started. But very few mothers who are single parents as a result of divorce or death would intentionally preplan to undergo parenting alone if there were other options.

Single women considering this alternative should think long and hard about the sacrifice involved and what the child will be missing without a present father in the home.

### Postmenopausal Women and Donor Eggs

Some of the most recent controversy about DI and egg donation involves its application to women who have passed the age of natural childbearing. Their bodies can still deliver a child, but once menopause has set in, they lose their egg-producing capacity. Even if they could still produce eggs, once a woman gets close to menopause, her eggs have aged and she runs a greater risk of genetic abnormalities for her child.

On the surface, she would seem to be an ideal candidate for egg donation. She has the experience of many years of life to give to a child, and it would seem arbitrary and perhaps even discriminatory to deny procreative liberty to someone simply because of age.

One of the earliest celebrated cases of so-called granny pregnancies occurred in 1994 in Italy when, through the use of egg donation, sixty-three-year-old Rosanna Della Corte gave birth to a child through the help of infertility specialist Dr. Severino Antinori. Della Corte wanted a second child when her seventeen-year-old son was killed in 1991 in a motorcycle accident. She received the eggs of an anonymous donor that were fertilized with her husband's sperm (who was also in his sixties), and she delivered Riccardo (also the name of her first son[29]) by C-section.

Although it is well documented that women in their fifties can deliver healthy children successfully, Della Corte in her sixties presented a bit more risk because of her age. In 2009, Della Corte had some interesting advice for a sixty-six-year-old mum-to-be in the UK. She said that sixty-six was too old; sixty-three should be the limit. About her own child, she had this to say: "I am a religious woman but I don't see how the Church could get involved—as far as I was concerned God had taken a child from me but God had also answered our prayers and given us another child."[30]

As a result of some of these successes and the ethical concerns they raise, the Italian national medical association issued guidelines that prohibit reproductive technologies from use by single women, lesbians, and postmenopausal women.[31] Similarly in Britain, no postmenopausal women may have access to assisted reproductive technology; Elizabeth Munro, the sixty-six-year-old cited above, received IVF treatment in Ukraine.[32] In France, Parliament restricted use of reproductive technologies to infertile, heterosexual couples of child-bearing age.[33]

Though it seems unlikely that many postmenopausal women would want to bear children, the ones who do present some ethical challenges. On the one hand, should society place a limit on the age at which a woman can have a child, given the long tradition of procreative liberty in the West and since society has not been willing to place a similar prohibition on men? On the other hand, is it fair to the children being born out of these arrangements to have parents who may not live long enough for them to finish their childhood and adolescence?

Though it may not be enforceable or wise to discourage this practice by law, certainly it is appropriate to use all means available to discourage the practice. Such older parents expose their children to a statistically greater risk of being orphaned. It may be that God in His wisdom instituted menopause in order to prevent people from having children past the age when they were generally able to care for and nurture them.

To be sure, many grandparents today are parenting a second generation of children for a variety of reasons. They are providing an essential rescue function. But that is very different from preplanning a "granny pregnancy" that may put the child at risk of being orphaned. At the least, clinics should be responsible and restrict their services to women of childbearing age. Using assisted reproductive technology to defy nature and overcome menopause is quite different from using it to overcome infertility in couples of childbearing age.

## DI and the Impact on the Marriage

One concern of using DI with infertile couples of childbearing age is that often the introduction of technology will produce tension and stress in the marriage. The husband is infertile, and a substitute is being sought for him. In many cases, he may have a feeling of failure and dispensability, similar to the instances of female infertility being remedied through egg donation or surrogate motherhood.

One spouse may feel anger toward the partner who is infertile, causing further tension in the home. These concerns of the adults can be addressed through counseling, and they need to be seriously considered by those contemplating DI or egg donation.

## EIGHT KIDS AT AGE 54

Karen Johnston is a mom of eight, is expecting two more on the way, is 54 years old, and she is postmenopausal. While Karen is too old to legally have IVF treatment in Britain, she found fertility clinics in the Czech Republic that agreed to IVF treatment and egg donation at her age. Also, the cost of the treatment was significantly lower than a fertility clinic in Britain would have been. Karen was brought up in a large family and knew from the beginning that she wanted a large family of her own, and she admits that she is addicted to having babies; she loves the feeling of being pregnant and she loves having babies around. The twins that Karen carries are from the second pregnancy from IVF and egg donation, both which she has had since going through menopause. While Karen admits the twins will be her last pregnancy, it seems if her body could keep going she would be happy to have another.

Source: Boudicca Fox-Leonard, "Why Having Eight Kids at 54 Isn't Enough for Me," *Mirror. co.uk News,* March 10, 2010, Mirror.co.uk.

## *DI and the Impact on the Child*

A second concern is the impact on the child. What does DI do to the sense of individual identity that the child develops? When, if at all, should the parents tell the child of his or her origins? If they choose not to tell, does this constitute an unjustifiable form of deception about the child's heritage? These are important questions, particularly since they involve the most important person in the matrix, the child produced by these arrangements.

One young man whose story is told in *The Genius Factory* had this to say after learning about his sperm donor dad: "And so now I have no father. My father—my mom's husband—isn't my father. My *real* father—the donor—isn't my father because all he did was donate sperm, which is not enough to make him a father. So nobody is my father."[34]

As more children of sperm donor–dads become aware of their heritage, people who are considering DI will have more information than previous generations. Some donor children seem fine with the arrangements, while others search for their fathers. The Donor Sibling Registry was begun by Wendy Kramer in 2000 to match offspring of donors to their donors or at least to their siblings. As of March 2010, the "DSR has helped connect more than 7,157 half-siblings (and/or donors) with each other. The total number of registrants, including donors, parents and donor conceived people, is currently at 26,845."[35]

Longitudinal studies are being conducted on children born of assisted arrangements such as surrogacy, for example, but it is still too early to tell what are the effects on the children. Of course, there are two different approaches to this lack of information. The first is to move ahead until the risks are proven, giving primacy to procreative liberty until harm is established. The second is to move more cautiously, waiting until harm is proven not to be occurring before moving forward more aggressively.

At present, the impact on the child is still an open question. It will likely take at least another decade until enough information is available to draw firm conclusions in this area. It may be that the impact on the children will parallel that of adoption, in which the results are mixed. Some children thrive in adoptive homes while others struggle. But it will be difficult to make any conclusions about the impact of ARTs on children until enough data has been amassed.

If, what, and when to tell the child about his or her genetic origins are not easy issues to address. Several of the donor-conceived children in David Plotz's *The Genius Factory: The Curious History of the Nobel Prize Sperm Bank* were not surprised that the man each thought was his/her father was, in fact, not the father. One mother, Beth, explained it this way to her ten-year-old daughter:

> She told Joy that her daddy was her daddy, but that she *also* had a "donor daddy," a special, very smart man who had helped her get born. . . . Joy wasn't surprised to learn she had a second father. "She loves her dad, but he is very different

from her," Beth told me. "I think it made sense to her that there could be this other father, too."[36]

Another donor-conceived child, Katrina Clark, expresses well the roller coaster of emotions in her *Washington Post* article, "My Father Was an Anonymous Sperm Donor":

When my mother eventually got married, I didn't get along with her husband. For so long, it had been just the two of us, my mom and I, and now I felt like the odd girl out. When she and I quarreled, this new man in our lives took to interjecting his opinion, and I didn't like that. One day, I lost my composure and screamed that he had no authority over me, that he wasn't my father—because I didn't have one.

That was when the emptiness came over me. I realized that I am, in a sense, a freak. I really, truly would never have a dad. I finally understood what it meant to be donor-conceived, and I hated it.[37]

We as a society do not know much about this social experiment called donor-conceived children. These two very different examples fit in a spectrum of the children's experiences. Parents struggle with whether or not to tell the child of his or her genetic origins, how much to tell, and when is the best time. Some may choose not to tell the children of their origins, but secrets have power, and tend to erode relationships.

Increasingly, though, with societal focus on the genetic basis of many diseases, it seems that not telling the child is less of an option than it was previously. Whenever the important information is conveyed, it needs to be done in terms the child can understand. This is a volatile subject, and parents need to be aware of this aspect—for themselves and their children. Such information can, but should not, be used as a weapon of shame toward the infertile spouse, or as an instrument to damage or sever the relationship between the child and the infertile spouse. This part of bearing donor-conceived children might not be addressed early in the process, for the object is usually "to have a baby." Long-term adverse ramifications may exist for the adults, but it should be underscored that the persons most greatly affected by these decisions are the children.

## Conclusion

Couples contemplating DI and egg donation should be very careful about employing these techniques given the biblical model for procreation and some of the unknowns about the donor(s) and the impact on the child. Single women should be even more cautious since rearing a child alone is extremely demanding and because Scripture suggests that children be born into a family with an involved father and mother, which is also in the child's best interest.

Of all the alternatives for procreation, it seems that the use of donor gametes would be best avoided. If other techniques that use the genetic material of the husband and wife cannot for some reason be utilized, other options such as embryo adoption or newborn/child adoption would be good considerations. In these, both parents share equally in the "otherness" of the child, and a child is rescued—benefits all around.

*Couples who use these procedures should be committed to giving every embryo created in the lab an opportunity for implantation and development.*

# CHAPTER SIX

# GIFT, ZIFT, and IVF

When James and Jill married ten years ago, children were not really a consideration. They were both on career tracks, and determined not to allow anything or anyone to inhibit their progress. That mind-set lasted four years, and for the past six years, they have been trying to conceive a child. Jill has even been known to list all the names she could find that begin with "J" as potential names of their children. Alas, there has been no pregnancy test with a "+" result thus far.

After years of frustration at trying to conceive a child naturally, they tried intrauterine insemination a number of times, each attempt ending up a failure. Uneasy about involving a third party by using donor sperm, they decided to explore some other options to have a baby by combining her egg and his sperm. Their obstetrician referred them to a clinic for assisted reproduction in their area. After an initial phone conversation, they made an appointment to meet with a nurse in the center, who would explain the available alternatives, the procedures involved, the advantages of each, and the costs involved.

### Getting the Facts

When they sat down with the center's nurse, Jill and James recounted briefly their story of infertility, how they had tried unsuccessfully both naturally and artificially, and how they now felt ready to consider entering the world of technologically assisted reproduction. They expressed concern that it would turn their lives upside down for the next few months and take them on an emotional and financial roller coaster ride like they had never experienced before, for they had seen this in the lives of two couples they knew.

The nurse explained that the clinic provided various reproductive services. Usually, the more complicated the procedure and the higher the rate of success, the more expensive it was likely to be. The clinic specialized in in vitro fertilization (IVF), but also occasionally did gamete intrafallopian transfer (GIFT) or zygote intrafallopian transfer (ZIFT). She explained that though there were some similarities among the procedures, the individual couple's specific situation affected the procedures recommended, as well as the rate of success.

She told them that these are medically very complicated procedures that sometimes involve outpatient surgery. When James asked about the center's success rate, she brought out a small stack of papers that the clinic had submitted to the Centers for Disease Control and Prevention (CDC).[1] She helped interpret the data for them and showed them that the center's success rate was consistent with the national averages for the various procedures, and in a few situations, better.

## Getting the Stats

As a result of the *Fertility Clinic Success Rate and Certification Act of 1992*, the collection of data from fertility centers in the United States is charged to the CDC, based in Atlanta, Georgia. The CDC posts success rates for different procedures from the reporting clinics, as well as national averages, on their website. The entry to the ART section is http://www.cdc.gov/ART/index.htm.[2] The ART cycles are described, and the pregnancy success rates are broken down in two ways: age of mother, and procedures done.

The most recent year as of this writing for which national statistics are available is 2007. In that year, 430 clinics reported that more than 99 percent of their procedures were IVF; GIFT and ZIFT were less than 1 percent, combined. In 63 percent of cases, intracytoplasmic sperm injection (ICSI) was used. The types of cycles reported included:[3]

*Fresh Embryos from Nondonor Eggs*—95,765 cycles for 2007

*Frozen Embryos from Nondonor Eggs*—20,544 embryos transferred in 2007

*Donor Eggs*—total of 15,953 cycles in 2007

The percentage of cycles resulting in pregnancy is higher than the percentage of cycles resulting in live births. Since live births are the goal, that is the data one needs to observe most closely. Generally speaking, the best success rates were obtained from women who were younger. The rates of pregnancy and live births per cycle decreased with increasing maternal age and nondonor eggs.

The highest success rate of live births per cycle was obtained with "Fresh Embryos" from donor eggs. Women of all ages were lumped into this statistic: 55 percent live birth rate. All other live births per cycle were lower; some, substantially so. The number of transferred embryos per cycle was between two and three.

It is important to note, also, that the majority of clinics reporting offered services to single women and gestational carriers. Therefore, these statistics represent more than heterosexual couples struggling with infertility. They include some fertile females without husbands (not separated out in the data), as well as fertile gestational carriers (less than 1 percent in 2007) who are seeking to bear children. These inclusions, particularly if substantial in number, can affect the overall data positively to produce higher rates of pregnancy or live births.

## *Jill's Part*

After being shown the data charts for that particular clinic, James and Jill asked specifically what was involved in each of the techniques offered. The nurse spelled out the processes involved with each technology and gave them estimates of the costs, but first she covered some basic information.

A cycle begins with the monitoring of developing follicles (maturing eggs) in the woman—usually when the woman begins taking fertility drugs to stimulate follicle production. Sometimes a medication is given to shut down the woman's system, before the fertility drugs are administered. The fertility drugs may include both oral and injected medications. The injected medications usually are given for about two weeks—daily. Both Jill and James could be trained to do this.

All the medications have expected effects and possible side effects. These range from menopausal symptoms (if her system is "shut down") to headaches, fatigue, and mood swings typical of menstrual cycles, but more pronounced, due to the increased number of follicles developing. Sometimes the "controlled ovarian stimulation" can lead to excessive fluid retention, and on occasion, serious health issues. This ovarian hyperstimulation can involve multiple organ systems—particularly heart, lungs, and kidneys—with rare deaths reported.

The retrieval (also called "harvesting") of the oocytes, or eggs, is done with ultrasound (usually transvaginal) guidance. The physician retrieves the eggs with a needle through the vaginal wall, guided by an ultrasound picture of the womb. This is usually done with conscious sedation. The experience sounds more painful and complicated than it typically is.

What is done next with the eggs depends on what procedure(s) the couple chooses. That choice depends on the particulars of their situation. Both GIFT and ZIFT require fallopian tubes to be open, not scarred or damaged.

In IVF, fertilization takes place in the petri dish, and the resulting embryo(s) are placed in the uterus. Therefore, the condition of the fallopian tubes is not of much concern. If Jill's fallopian tubes are not damaged, she produces eggs normally, and James's sperm is acceptable in terms of their number, their ability to swim, and their ability to penetrate the egg, the couple could be eligible for any of the three procedures, but IVF will most likely be the one that is offered. This is because both GIFT and ZIFT involve a second procedure, and add thousands of dollars to the cost.

### James's Part

The nurse explained James's role at this point. "We need a sperm sample from you. I know this can be awkward, but here's how it works. We give you a sterile cup, put you in the men's room, and you give us a sperm sample through masturbation. Then we'll have all the raw material we need to conceive a baby."

What sounds simple when the nurse explained it to James is actually a bit more complicated. The nurse didn't include the part about the pornographic movies and magazines provided in the room where James will produce his sample. In most cases the clinic treats the sperm sample as something that simply has to be done, and considers the use of porn to arouse the man as part of the process. In our view, the sample should be procured by husband and wife together, so as to avoid accommodating pornography and the lust that inevitably occurs when sperm samples are obtained. Think about this from Jill's perspective—would she really want her husband to be contemplating the women in the pictures while attempting to fertilize her eggs?

## Next Steps

The nurse continued. "James, your sperm is treated in our lab to make it best prepared to fertilize one of Jill's eggs. With GIFT, the sperm and some of the eggs are put together in a catheter in our lab but kept separate by a divider so they won't fertilize in the catheter. Then, the procedure gets a bit complicated again.

"The eggs and sperm are returned to Jill's fallopian tubes, but this time it does take that minor surgical procedure I mentioned earlier called laparoscopy. This requires anesthesia and you will need to drive Jill home from the clinic after it's done. The next step is waiting for your sperm to fertilize one of her eggs, and if all goes according to plan, you'll be pregnant. You may end up being pregnant with more than one baby. That is not an uncommon occurrence. In fact, if you see a woman with twins, or especially triplets, you can almost bet that she conceived them through some form of ART.

## In Vitro

"IVF is our most common means of helping couples become pregnant. We offer several options for you to maximize your efforts to have a baby. Retrieving the eggs is the hardest and most expensive part of the process. With the stimulation of the ovaries by the drugs, Jill may produce, and we will retrieve, more eggs than would be needed for one cycle. It would be a shame to throw away the eggs that we don't use. So we suggest that you let us fertilize the leftover eggs in the lab and store the embryos for you in case you need them later. Getting pregnant by GIFT is not a sure thing, and the embryos of ZIFT or IVF don't always implant, so you can think of this as a kind of insurance. You will have some embryos in storage that we can implant in Jill if the first cycle doesn't produce a pregnancy.

## What about Multiples?

"Another service I need to mention is offered in case you develop a multiple pregnancy. If you only want one baby, or could maybe handle two, but you are pregnant with three, and you think that three babies will be too much for you either to carry and deliver or rear, we can refer you to physicians in our community who offer what is called 'selective termination.' They have a good track record of reducing the number you are carrying in this pregnancy without risking the health of the remaining babies. You may not be interested in that, but some couples are, and I wanted you to know about it.[4]

## ZIFT

"If you are not a good candidate for GIFT, and do not wish to go the IVF route, we recommend that you think about trying ZIFT. That stands for zygote intrafallopian transfer. We can use this when there is no male infertility factor, and when Jane's fallopian tubes are in relatively good condition. We retrieve the eggs in the same way, fertilize them in the lab as with IVF, but we transfer the embryos to Jane's fallopian tubes, usually within twenty-four to forty-eight hours of fertilization. We do this because the success rate is higher if the embryos are placed in the tubes. Reinserting the embryos does require minor surgery—laparoscopy—unfortunately. As with GIFT and IVF, you can store the remaining embryos for later use. Storing the embryos keeps the cost down and reduces the wear and tear on Jane's body that egg retrieval involves.

## The Cost

"Now I'm sure you're interested in the costs of all these procedures. The costs vary depending on how much medication Jane needs to produce the eggs in her cycle. Other components of cost include the process of egg retrieval, embryo transfer, and other options you might use, like ICSI or gamete (egg or sperm) donation. Procedures that involve laparoscopy are more expensive. If you want some embryos stored for later use, that is an extra expense, too. I don't know what your insurance covers, but I do know that some insurance companies cover at least part of the cost.[5] We require two deposits, one up front

## SURROGATE HANDS OVER CHILD AFTER IVF MISTAKE

Sometimes mistakes made in infertility clinics actually bring out the best in people. At a Toledo, Ohio, IVF clinic, Carolyn Savage became an "accidental surrogate," giving birth to a child who she immediately gave up upon birth. Savage had been accidently implanted with embryos belonging to another couple, Shannon and Paul Morell. The Morells had embryos in storage when they came to the clinic to have them implanted in order to try for their third child. But the clinic called with the news that their embryos had been thawed and transferred mistakenly to Savage. Savage had the choice to end the pregnancy or carry the child to term and hand him/her over to the Morells. She chose to endure the pregnancy and give up the baby to the Morells. The couples met during the pregnancy and became friends, and the Morells gave the child the middle name of Savage.

Source: "Accidental Surrogate Hands Baby Over after IVF Mistake," Telegraph, May 10, 2010, http://www.telegraph.co.uk/news/worldnews/northamerica/usa/7703470/Accidental-surrogate-hands-over-baby-after-IVF-mistake.html.

and a second one just prior to your egg retrieval procedure. Any balance left over must be settled at the end of the process."

### Much to Think About

James and Jill left the clinic, stunned. They barely made it into the car before James exploded, "Fifteen thousand dollars? The round figure is fifteen thousand dollars?!"

"And that is with *our* gametes," responded Jill. "I remember our chemistry professor in college told us how little our bodies were worth in terms of the chemicals involved. Apparently he never needed IVF!"

"Fifteen thousand dollars," mused James, "for a *try* at getting pregnant: no guarantees. We can hope we won't need egg donation!"

With that in mind, James and Jill changed their dinner plans. Instead of the romantic spot across town, they opted for soup and sandwich at a nearby gourmet-to-go spot. Enjoying their meal at their own table, they began to talk about their experience at the clinic. There was so much to consider . . .

## Moral Evaluation of GIFT, IVF, and ZIFT

In most cases, use of these technologies does not involve a third party contributor, since the couple involved desires to have a child from their own genetic materials. Thus there would be no concern about violating the creation model for procreation outlined in chapter 2. Additionally, the use of sperm or egg donors is covered in the previous chapter, and will not be repeated here.

For those who believe that personhood begins at conception, GIFT, ZIFT, and IVF have two potential moral difficulties. It is certainly better for the couple who chooses to use either of these procedures to enter into them aware of the possible problem areas. Many couples do not become aware of the potential problems until after they are deeply involved in the process, and at times, after they are pregnant and thinking that the process is over. This leaves them with some agonizing decisions to make.

### *Leftover Embryos*

The first moral problem area, in the case of ZIFT or IVF, is how many eggs to fertilize. Some countries have laws that mandate that clinics can only fertilize the number of eggs they will implant.[6] That is to say, there are no "leftovers"—the term given to embryos that will not be implanted in a given cycle. These are frozen in liquid nitrogen and kept until a disposition is made. In the United States, we have no laws limiting the number of eggs fertilized per ART cycle, which has resulted in many embryos being kept frozen year after year.

This is the critical part of the first moral problem area: leftover embryos. By April 2002, the United States had nearly 400,000 frozen "leftover" embryos.[7] The disposition of these lies properly in the hands of their parents, although many are left for years in the deep cold, for which a maintenance fee—not insignificant—is charged.

This difficulty is created by the cost of the procedures and their modest success rate. Since egg retrieval is so expensive and so inconvenient, physicians attempt to have the woman produce, and then they harvest as many eggs as possible in one cycle. The eggs are all fertilized at the same time, and some embryos implanted.

As the nurse mentioned to James and Jill, leftover embryos are a kind of insurance in case pregnancy is not achieved—the couple can simply thaw out embryos that are in storage instead of starting an expensive process over again. But if they achieve all their goals for having children and have embryos left over, what to do with those embryos that they no longer intend to use is a very difficult moral issue to resolve.

In the wake of the 2009 "Octomom" affair (Nadya Suleman was thirty-three years of age and already had six children when she gave birth to octuplets), the American Society for Reproductive Medicine (ASRM) and the Society for Assisted Reproductive Technology (SART) issued new recommendations for numbers of embryos to be implanted. These depend on the age of the woman involved, and the stage of the embryos. The very early stage embryos have a lower chance of implanting, so there is some leeway with these. Once the embryo reaches blastocyst stage (five days after fertilization), implantation is more likely. For women at different ages, here are the recommendations of number of embryos and their stages:

*Under 35 years*—not more than two should be implanted; transfer of a single embryo should be considered

*35–37 years*—not more than three early stage, or two blastocyst stage embryos

*38–40 years*—three to four early stage; two to three blastocyst stage, depending on woman's prognosis

*41–42 years*—no more than five earlier stage, or three blastocyst stage embryos

The ASRM and SART deemed the data for older mothers as insufficient for recommendations regarding number of embryos to be implanted.[8] Embryos not implanted are frozen and kept in storage should they be needed if the woman does not become pregnant with the first attempt at implantation.

Like IVF, GIFT includes hormonal stimulation for oocyte (egg) production. Unlike IVF, after egg retrieval, GIFT requires a laparoscopy (minor surgery), during which the woman's eggs and her husband's sperm are inserted into her fallopian tube. It is in the fallopian tube that fertilization usually takes place, and as in ZIFT, GIFT requires at least one patent (open) fallopian tube. Whereas in IVF, fertilization can be visually confirmed, fertilization in GIFT is unseen.

### Extra Eggs

The possibility for a multiple pregnancy with GIFT, as with any ART, is a concern. For that reason, the number of eggs transferred may be limited. What is done with the remaining harvested eggs? If the couple consents, the remaining eggs may be fertilized, and the embryos frozen for future use. (Egg freezing at this time is still considered experimental, and the availability of this option is increasing but not yet widespread.) Should pregnancy not occur, the couple could then thaw the remaining embryos and attempt implantation again. This scenario would obviate a second egg retrieval, but hormonal preparation of the woman's uterus would have to be done. The medications used would be less in amount and therefore not as costly than that for egg retrieval.

Most clinics assume that the couple will want to avoid starting over if the first attempt at achieving pregnancy fails, and would recommend freezing leftover embryos. But trying to make the process less medically and financially complicated has actually made it more ethically complicated for the couple who holds that personhood begins at conception. Of course, for the couple who believes that the unborn acquires personhood at some point after conception, this is not a problem. But for the Christian couple who is trying to be consistent with Scripture in their entire approach to these reproductive technologies, what to do with leftover embryos presents a significant problem.

### Personhood of the Embryo

The reason this is a problem is that embryos are persons, deserving of full human rights. They are not potential persons, a concept that itself is problematic: one either is a person or one is not a person. To speak of a potential person is philosophically absurd, because personhood is not a degreed property.[9] What one normally means by using that imprecise term is that the embryo (and fetus also) is a person with the potential to become a full grown adult. It is better to say that the embryo is a "person with potential."

## What about the Extra Embryos?

The disposition of excess or "leftover" embryos is a complicated dilemma. The American Society for Reproductive Medicine (ASRM) reports that, from 1985 through the year 2006, "almost 500,000 babies have been born in the United States as a result of reported Assisted Reproductive Technology procedures (IVF, GIFT, ZIFT, and combination procedures)."[10] This is remarkable, but pales in comparison to the number of embryos not implanted: "As of April 11, 2002, a total of 396,526 embryos have been placed in storage in the United States."[11] From these numbers, and the more than four years that separate them, it appears that for every child born through ART in the United States, another embryo is in frozen storage.

What happens to these embryos in storage? The decision may be complicated, as the story of Pam and Kai Madsen exemplifies. She produced a substantial number of eggs through hormonal stimulation, and excess embryos were stored. Thirteen years after the birth of their second child, the Madsens still had four embryos in storage. In the *60 Minutes* episode where their story was told in 2006,

## IVF AND STILLBIRTH

A study published in the journal *Human Reproduction* claims that women who have IVF or ICSI are four times more likely to have a stillborn baby than those who conceive without fertility treatments. The lead researcher of the study, Kirsten Wisborg, acknowledges that the risk of stillbirth is still very low for women who have fertility treatments and that the ultimate cause of the increased risk is still undetermined. In the study researchers followed over twenty thousand pregnancies but determined that the evidence was insufficient for determining what is causing the increased risk in women who have IVF or ICSI. Researchers recognize the increased risk may be due to the nature of the fertility treatment, the physiology of parents who typically have trouble conceiving, or to other unknown factors.

Source: Sarah Boseley, "Still Births Four Times More Likely with IVF," Feb. 23, 2010, guardian.co.uk.

the Madsens elucidated five choices they had regarding the frozen embryos:

> "Well, one, we could have used them to have a third child, the potential of a third child. We could have destroyed them, not used them and . . . have them thawed and put away. We could have donated them to another couple who's having reproductive difficulties and wants to have a baby. We could continue to do nothing. Or we could donate them to medical research," Pam explains.[12]

### Some Options

It is useful to take a closer look at these possibilities.

1. Implantation—this would mean hormonal treatment to ready her womb, and the potential addition of a child/children to their family, depending on the outcome of the procedure.
2. Destruction of the embryos—have the embryos thawed and

"put away": this would mean disposed of as biological waste, since the embryos will die if not implanted.

3. Donate them to another infertile couple—this is also termed "embryo adoption." Donations like this would be seen as the practical, though not legal, equivalent of adoption. The couple would simply put embryos, not newborn babies, up for "adoption." Embryo donation is not anywhere near as complicated legally as formal adoption, and the infertile couple gets the experience of carrying and delivering their child—if pregnancy occurs. It should be noted that in embryo adoption, there is no guarantee of the birth of a child.

4. "Do nothing"—means continuing to pay a storage fee for the frozen embryos. It also means staying in touch with the clinic/lab where these are stored. It should be noted that embryo storage facilities are allowed to destroy embryos (by thawing and disposal only—no transfer to another couple or use in research) if the embryos have been abandoned. Abandonment of embryos means the clinic and the couple whose embryo(s) are being stored have had no contact for five years, despite specific attempts by the clinic to reach them by mail or telephone, and "no written instruction from the couple exists concerning disposition."[13]

5. Donate embryos for research—which will normally involve their eventual discard or destruction.

## The Embryo as "Waste"

The practice of discarding embryos is problematic for couples who hold that personhood begins at conception. *Throwing away embryos that a couple does not plan to use is morally no different from abortion at any point during the pregnancy.* Only the location of the unborn child and its stage of development are different. Since the embryo has all the capacities to mature into a fully grown adult from the point of conception, needing only the proper environment in which to develop, then the point at which it is destroyed and discarded is irrelevant. A person with a unique genetic endowment and with full potential to become a fully grown adult human being has been destroyed.

Some have further lamented the fact that human embryos are being treated as the equivalent of "industrial waste," a by-product of the procedure that is thrown out when no longer needed.[14] Experimenting on embryos does not seem to be morally different, since the experiment will usually result in the destruction or deformation of the embryo, and since the embryos that do survive the experiments are usually discarded after they are no longer useful for research.

## Two Complex Cases

Leftover embryos raise more than complicated moral problems; there are some legal problems that would have tested the wisdom of Solomon. Two extraordinary cases that attracted worldwide attention illustrate the myriad of legal problems that are possible when couples have embryos left in storage.

**Mario and Elsa Rios:** In 1981, embryos left in storage were orphaned, leaving behind a tangle of legal complications. Mario and Elsa Rios were a wealthy California couple who had no heirs to their sizeable estate. They traveled to Australia to have IVF performed. In the early days of these procedures, some of the pioneering work was done in England and Australia, which is why they sought out Australian specialists.

Elsa had several eggs of her own fertilized with donor sperm in the lab. A number of embryos were implanted and two were frozen and kept in storage for later use if necessary. The first round of embryos failed to implant. Mario and Elsa returned to California, presumably planning to visit Australia again and have the remaining two embryos implanted. However, before they could get back to Australia, they were both killed in a plane crash in South America.

Their deaths left the Australian infertility clinic that had the embryos in storage with some difficult problems. Australian law had not yet addressed situations like these, so there were no legal guidelines available to the clinic. What were they to do with the Rioses' embryos?

No doubt there was a long line of potential surrogate mothers waiting to be implanted with those embryos in order to stake a claim to part or all of the Rioses' estate. A nationally appointed committee looked into the matter and recommended that the embryos be destroyed, thereby solving the problem by eliminating it. The Australian government agreed.

But the state of Victoria, in which the clinic was located, saw it differently, and mandated that the embryos be implanted in a surrogate mother, then placed for adoption. That created legal nightmares about the distribution of the Rioses' estate. Should the surrogates be entitled to any share of the estate for carrying the embryos? Should the adoptive parents be entitled to child support, or a sizeable share of the estate to pay for the children's additional expenses such as college? Or should the estate be divided equally among the children born of these surrogates? It is not hard to imagine these surrogates, once pregnant, being in a strong position to demand whatever they wanted out of the Rios estate.

At this point the attorney for the Rioses' estate stepped in and insisted that the embryos could not be heirs under American law because donor sperm, not Mr. Rios's, was used to fertilize the eggs. But normally donor sperm is used with the presumption that the man married to the woman who gives birth to the child is the legal father. That is, sperm donors are not presumed to have paternal rights to the child born from their sperm.

The clinic attempted to implant the embryos in a surrogate, but when that failed, there was no longer a problem that needed resolution.[15]

**Junior and Mary Sue Davis:** A second remarkable case involved frozen embryos as the subject of a custody dispute. Unlike the Rios case, this one required court intervention to resolve the dispute. Junior and Mary Sue Davis were a Tennessee couple who underwent

IVF six different times, and had seven embryos left in storage at the end of all their attempts. They divorced, leaving the status of the left-over embryos in legal limbo. Mary Sue wanted the embryos implanted in her in order to have a child. Junior Davis wanted them to be left in storage.

The first problem that the courts faced was deciding whether the embryos were property, to be divided equally, or children, to be awarded based on what would be in their best interests. The court had to determine whether this was a property or custody dispute. The trial court decided that they were children and awarded them to Mary Sue. Since she wanted them implanted, born, and raised, the court ruled that that course of action constituted their best interests.

In 1990, the appeals court reversed that decision, awarding both parties an equal voice in the embryos' future.[16] This decision was based on the principle of privacy, that no one should be forced to become a parent against one's will, as Junior Davis would have been had the lower court's decision been allowed to stand. In other words, the right to procreate also includes a right not to procreate, according to one's choice.

In 1992, the Tennessee Supreme Court essentially upheld the decision of the court of appeals. However, by the time the Supreme Court decision came around, Mary Sue had remarried and wished to donate the embryos rather than have them implanted in her. These were but the beginning of the embryo disputes.[17]

## Cryopreservation

Is there a viable alternative to storing embryos? The most obvious alternative to discarding the embryos would be to store the woman's eggs prior to fertilization in the lab. That way, eggs, not embryos, are being stored. The couple has eggs left over to use again in the future, avoiding the entire process of egg retrieval, while at the same time, not destroying and discarding embryonic human persons.

It needs to be noted that the use of cryopreserved eggs necessitates the use of ICSI (intracytoplasmic sperm injection) in attempting fertilization, based on technical considerations alone. Egg freezing (oocyte cryopreservation) is a recent technological development, and currently labeled "experimental" by the ASRM. The first birth from a previously frozen egg occurred in 1986; by 2004, about a hundred children had been born from cryopreserved eggs.[18] However, though still experimental, egg freezing may be becoming a more viable alternative.

Still, since the long-term risks (to the babies born) of egg freezing are unknown at present, we cannot at this time recommend it. Because of the way in which eggs are treated in order to be frozen, ICSI is the only methodology available to fertilize them. This, of course, adds another cost to the IVF undertaking.

## EGG FREEZING

In 2004 the American Society for Reproductive Medicine (ASRM) established that egg freezing is an experimental procedure. ASRM concluded that doctors must obtain permission from a review board before offering to do the procedure, and patients must be informed that the medical procedure is not established. However, while some doctors are aligned with ASRM's view, other physicians argue that babies born from frozen-egg embryos are just as healthy as babies born from natural procedures. In fact, some of these doctors argue that ASRM was inconsistent to label egg-freezing "experimental" because many other reproductive technologies, such as screening embryos for abnormalities and injecting sperm into eggs, were never labeled such but were just as informal. The aim of freezing eggs is to allow women who are aging to not feel the pressure to have children quickly if they are not ready, but to have the option of waiting until they are ready. But doctors now argue that there may be good reason for women to drop their guards and consider the possibility of freezing their eggs.

Source: Sarah Elizabeth Richards, "Is Egg Freezing Unfairly Marginalized?" *Slate*, March 15, 2010, Slate.com.

## A Natural Death

A second alternative that some couples have contemplated is not intentionally discarding the embryos, but allowing them to die a natural death in the lab. They reason that it is parallel to a miscarriage, only it happens in the lab and not in the body. During a miscarriage, the fetus dies a natural death, and the corpse is extracted surgically and discarded, or it is expelled naturally from the body if it occurs at a very early stage of the pregnancy.

Many miscarriages occur prior to implantation, when the embryo fails to attach to the woman's uterine wall. Roughly half of all conceptions miscarry in this way, and thus many embryonic persons who are successfully conceived die a natural death at a very early phase of pregnancy. Thus, those who suggest this alternative insist that they are simply allowing something to happen in the lab that happens frequently in the body. Thus they would say that allowing embryos to die a natural death is more akin to a miscarriage than to an intentional abortion.

However, there is a morally significant difference besides location between a miscarriage and allowing embryos in storage to die natural deaths. Most miscarriages cannot be prevented; indeed, in most cases, no one fully understands why they occur. Many early miscarriages, those that happen prior to implantation, along with other later term miscarriages, are a mystery to physicians, leaving them baffled for an explanation as to why a particular pregnancy did not make it to term. In many cases, there is not much they can do to prevent future miscarriages.

Of course, some miscarriages can be traced to deformities in the fetus or problems in the woman's reproductive system. But a great many miscarriages appear to be random, spontaneous occurrences. Although a significant number of embryos do not survive the thawing process, the intentional destruction of laboratory-stored embryos is easily prevented. Instead of being thawed and destroyed, those that survive the thawing process could be implanted.

In medicine generally, it is certainly justifiable to allow some-one to die a natural death when it cannot be prevented. But to al-low someone to die from an easily preventable disease or condition is morally very problematic, and people who allow others to die natural deaths in this way are doing the moral equivalent of killing them. For example, though there may be some technical distinctions,[19] when parents, for whatever reason, refuse treatment for a child suffering from meningitis, which is easily treatable with antibiotics, society is morally outraged, and properly so. Many would say that the parents are, for all practical purposes, killing the child. In the same way, al-lowing embryos to be thawed with no intent to implant them is the moral equivalent of killing them, since their natural death is easily preventable.

### When Personhood Begins

One option of what to do with extra embryos is to hold the position that personhood begins at implantation, not conception.[20] This ap-proach, which has been adopted by both the American College of Ob-stetricians and Gynecologists (ACOG) and ASRM, has strong appeal for many.

The average person has a difficult time seeing how an embryo in a petri dish in the lab can be the moral equivalent of a baby growing in a mother's womb. Embryos in the lab seem so clinical and detached from a mother in whom they are developing, that it is hard to see how they can be persons. In addition, they cannot, at least for now, grow or develop outside the womb. Thus the uterine environment is indis-pensible for the embryo to develop fully.

The problem with this shift in one's view of when personhood be-gins is that there is no *essential* difference between the embryo in the lab and one that has been implanted in a woman's womb. The only difference is one of location, and location is unrelated to the essence of what the embryo is. The fact that the embryo's capacities cannot yet develop in certain locations is irrelevant to the fact that he/she still has all the capacities necessary to develop into a full adult from the moment of conception onward.

By analogy, almost everyone agrees that there is no essential difference between an unborn child one day before birth and a baby one day after birth. The only difference is one of location and dependence, the latter meaning that the baby is dependent on its mother in a different way than when it was in utero. Location by itself does not make a morally significant difference when it comes to the essential nature of the unborn child.

## Embryo Donation

Another alternative is to give the embryos away to another infertile couple. Donating the embryos is certainly a possibility that is morally different from discarding them, but many people are uncomfortable with the idea of donating their embryos to another couple. The notion of another couple, not to mention one they do not know, rearing a child that is the combination of their genetic materials and may even look like one or the other of them, can be very unsettling. As one person who was contemplating embryo donation put it, "I don't want my progeny running around all over the country without my knowledge!"

This uncomfortable feeling is often more intense when the couple realizes that they have not one, but a number of embryos in storage, all of which would need to be donated to keep from having to destroy them. Even though donation does not involve discarding the leftover embryos, and is more ethically acceptable, doing so is emotionally difficult to accept for many couples.

But if the couple is unable to implant the remaining embryos themselves, then putting them up for adoption may be the only morally acceptable option available to them.

Of course, the couple can always choose to implant the remaining embryos themselves, and consider any children born to be gifts from God. But for the family with twins or triplets from IVF, they may reasonably consider their childbearing days to be over. It may be medically

## EMBRYO ADOPTION OVERSEAS

The practice of embryo adoption, also known as embryo donation, is on the rise in India. Embryo adoption gives women who are
infertile or who have already gone through menopause the ability
to experience motherhood completely—pregnancy and all. With
injections and medication, a woman's uterus can be made to carry
and sustain a child. Patricia Bohanon, 51, is one client of the Malpani
Infertility Clinic in Mumbai. Patricia chose the clinic after considering numerous options for adoption, both traditional adoption and
embryo adoption. In the end, she found that an embryo adoption
through the Malpani Infertility Clinic would be about a fourth the
cost of an embryo adoption from other clinics around the world and
would be easier than adopting a child traditionally.

Source: Malathy Iyer, "Embryo Adoption Is Latest Trend," *The Times of India*, Feb. 12, 2010,
timesofindia.indiatimes.com.

possible, but may put them at risk of having a much larger family than
they had planned.

What does seem clear is that any option for the disposition of leftover embryos that involves their discard or destruction is the moral
equivalent of abortion and is not consistent with the biblical notion
that the unborn is a person from conception forward. At the least,
*a couple contemplating IVF should be committed to the principle that
every embryo created in the lab deserves to be implanted and is owed
an opportunity to mature into a newborn baby.* If the couple is not
comfortable with such an arrangement, they ought to think seriously
about the wisdom of going forward with IVF.

### Prevent the Conundrum

The most prudent course for a couple to follow in IVF procedures is to
avoid having leftover embryos. This can and does occasionally happen by chance, that is, if the couple actually uses all the embryos that
are produced in the lab through their sperm and eggs. The couple
should inform the clinic of their views concerning when personhood

begins, and tell them that they want to do whatever is possible to avoid having leftover embryos.

One way to work this out is for the clinic to harvest a sufficient number of eggs for only one round of embryo implants. That is, the number of eggs to be harvested depends on the number of embryos that the couple wants implanted at any one time. Often some of the eggs do not fertilize in the lab, so it may be prudent to allow for some attrition in the process. But to be perfectly safe, the couple may insist that all the eggs that are harvested be fertilized and eventually implanted. Up to three embryos are usually implanted. This scenario may mean that fewer eggs will be retrieved and fertilized; should the eggs fail to be fertilized, or the transferred embryos fail to develop, then the couple would be faced with another cycle of egg retrieval and fertilization in the lab.

This choice will likely significantly increase the cost as well as the risk of ovarian hyperstimulation, should the couple elect to continue trying to become pregnant with one of these procedures. Should the couple not wish to undertake this financial risk of starting over and conduct IVF according to the normal practice, they should be prepared to either implant or donate to another couple any remaining embryos when they have finished with IVF.

Many couples will not be comfortable with these constraints that could further drive up the costs of achieving pregnancy. So in an effort to keep the costs down, they go ahead and have harvested and fertilized as many eggs as can be retrieved, and store the excess embryos.

But for the couple who holds that human personhood begins at conception, doing so is morally problematic. Should they expose their offspring, their embryos, to the perils of freezing and thawing, since by so doing, the embryos may well not survive? Since the physicians cannot predict how many eggs they will successfully retrieve or how many will fertilize, it may not be technologically feasible to operate within these limits. If it is inevitable that a couple will have leftover embryos, and if they are unwilling to implant or donate those that remain, then this raises serious questions about the moral acceptability of these techniques.

If personhood begins at conception and if location of the embryos is not relevant to their personhood, then discarding leftover embryos is problematic. The couple should be prepared to work within limits that do not produce leftovers, or be prepared to either have implanted those that remain after they achieve pregnancy, or donate them to other infertile couples.

Donation of embryos can be seen as parallel to adoption, a rescue operation that is the exception to the general rule of parents keeping their children. Scripture clearly allows adoption and does not view it as a violation of the creation model for procreation, but rather as heroic rescue of the vulnerable. The only difference is the time at which the rescue takes place, prior to implantation instead of at birth.

It may be that this quandary will be resolved when the procedure of egg freezing and thawing is perfected. Discarding leftover, unfertilized eggs does not have the moral implications of discarding embryos, although leftover unfertilized eggs will most likely bring a whole new set of ethical conundra to the fore.[21] Egg freezing is used today with women who must postpone childbearing due to some reason, such as cancer treatments, that produce the onset of menopause. A woman in such a situation may be able to store a harvest of eggs until she is healthy and ready to start a family.

### Selective Termination

A second and even more troubling ethical issue in these techniques results not from the failure of the embryo implants but from their successes. Pregnancies of multiples are not uncommon with these technologies. In fact, if a family has fraternal twins or especially triplets, chances are good that they came from use of one of these techniques, although certainly not all twins or triplets are so conceived.

In many cases, couples are so eager to have a child that when they learn they are finally pregnant it matters little how many children they have. But some couples are clearly distressed with pregnancies of multiples, due to the higher risk involved, and/or because they did not want as many children as the woman is carrying. Sometimes more embryos will implant than the woman can safely carry to term.

When either of these situations occur, the clinics will suggest what is called a "reduction" in the number of pregnancies the woman is carrying. It is also called "selective termination." The clinic normally does not perform the reduction but will refer the couple to a practitioner in the local area who will perform the selective abortion.

In this procedure, a physician uses a needle that is inserted into the woman's abdominal wall and guided by ultrasound to the embryos or fetuses to be eliminated. A saline solution of potassium chloride is injected into the fetus(es) to be destroyed, and if they have developed to the point at which the heart can be detected by ultrasound, then the injection is made directly into the heart. The injection kills the developing embryo. It is the essential equivalent of saline abortions that are often used for later term abortions.

### Ethical Considerations of Reduction

For the couple who holds that personhood begins at conception, these "reductions" are very problematic. There is no morally significant difference between these reductions and abortion for unwanted pregnancies.

In fact, these reductions are ethically more troubling than ordinary abortions. That is not to say that the embryos that are reduced are any less persons than fetuses that are aborted or that abortions for birth control reasons are somehow justifiable. With abortion for family planning reasons, a pregnancy that was not intended is terminated. (Though it is true that by virtue of having sex, the couple knew that pregnancy was a possible outcome, it was nevertheless unplanned and accidental.) This is particularly so if reasonable birth control measures were taken and they failed, and to be clear, we are not suggesting that abortion is justified for failure of birth control measures.

But with a reduction, the embryos were *deliberately* implanted in the woman. The couple consented to the implanted embryos, knowing from the start that each one might "take" (and even divide, yielding more embryos than were implanted) and develop in the uterus. There is a degree of intentionality in these techniques that is not a part of abortions with unplanned pregnancies. Embryonic life is deliberately—not accidently—created in the lab and intentionally implanted in the woman. This makes pregnancy reduction in these cases seem more callous and less respectful of developing personhood than with ordinary abortions. To deliberately create human life, implant it in the uterus where it can grow, and then terminate it because the couple does not want that many children is very troubling when it comes to society's respect for the life it is intentionally creating.

Reductions raise complicated questions about the details involved in carrying them out. For example, which embryos are terminated? On what basis is that decision made? And perhaps most importantly, who makes the decision? A close friend recalls going through GIFT and conceiving triplets, after already having one child. This gave them a total of four children, clearly more than they had anticipated and originally wanted. Having this many children would significantly stretch them financially. The temptation to undergo a reduction was strong. But they continued all of the pregnancies and even though it was physically very taxing on the woman (she was in a wheelchair for the last three months until delivery, and delivered over a month early) and very stressful to have three newborns at the same time, they are glad they made the decision they did.

After the triplets were born, one of the man's colleagues at work was in the middle of IVF with his wife. They too had conceived triplets, and were seriously contemplating a reduction. The two men talked and my friend explained that they were offered the same opportunity by their clinic. But after the children were born, in thinking back on considering reduction, he saw his children's faces, not just clinically detached embryos. He admitted that it was difficult to imagine which one of the three children would have been terminated in the reduction, or how they would have made that choice.

After realizing that these were persons who were growing in his wife's uterus, the colleague revealed that they had decided to continue all three pregnancies.

These are simply agonizing decisions even for couples who hold that abortion is justifiable. They are decisions that can almost always be avoided with proper planning, by simply limiting the number of embryos implanted to the number that the woman can safely carry or the number of children the couple wishes to rear.

## More to Consider

In cases in which the woman's life is endangered due to carrying the pregnancies, it may be justifiable to abort one of the pregnancies in order to save the mother's life. That is not because the mother's life is any more valuable than the unborn children she is carrying, but because if the mother dies, so will all of the children she is carrying. So it is not trading one life for another, but one life for two or perhaps three.

In some cases a physician will propose a reduction in order to safeguard the lives and health of the other fetuses the mother is carrying. For example, if by carrying four fetuses as long as she can, she runs the risk of delivering prematurely, and may seriously compromise the health and even the lives of the children who have been delivered early. The couple should be very careful about reducing the number of pregnancies in order to avoid the health problems that come with premature delivery.

We view it as very problematic that the life or lives of fetuses would be taken in order to safeguard the health of the other fetuses. We see this as compounding a previous error in judgment in the number of embryos implanted. In addition, we would weigh life more heavily than health and would opt for managing the pregnancy carefully and dealing with any problems from premature delivery, as opposed to eliminating one or more of the pregnancies.

It is true that four or more pregnancies does increase the risk of health problems due to prematurity. But there are numerous anecdotal cases in which multiple pregnancies are delivered successfully. In our view, it is not justifiable to do evil (terminate a pregnancy) in order to accomplish a good (safeguarding the life/health of the other fetuses). Again, with proper planning at the beginning of the procedure, this kind of difficult decision can be avoided.

A window into selective reduction is provided by a tragedy in Florida. A woman had conceived twins through in vitro fertilization: a boy and a girl. The male appeared to have Down syndrome, and perhaps a heart defect. The woman was advised that "selective termination was an option,"[22] and proceeded to have that done, at approximately sixteen weeks gestation. A mistake was made: the female fetus was selectively terminated instead. The physician who made the mistake lost his license, and the woman who conceived twins through IVF ultimately had both children terminated.

How commonly does such an error occur?

Dr. Mark Evans, a New York ob-gyn and geneticist who pioneered the procedure, said in a phone interview Monday he has not in twenty-five years heard of another case in which the wrong twin or fetus was terminated.

While records are not kept on how often the procedure is performed nationally, Evans said it requires significant expertise that few physicians possess.

"In my hands, it's not complicated because I do it every day of the week," said Evans, noting that half of his patients, including some from Florida, travel by plane to his Manhattan office, Comprehensive Genetics.[23]

The way to avoid the agonizing dilemma created by the prospect of a pregnancy reduction is to limit the number of embryos that are transferred from the start. The couple should insist that the number of embryos being transferred

1. be no more than the woman can safely carry to term; and
2. be only as many as they are willing to rear.

They need to seriously consider the possibility of rearing twins or even triplets, if they plan to have more than two embryos transferred. In 2003, it was not uncommon to transfer three or four embryos, and the rate of triplets (or greater multiples) at birth ranged from 2.8 to 6.4 percent.[24] By 2008, the practice of embryo transfer had changed. In that year, the average number of embryos transferred was much closer to two, and the resulting percentage of triplets or greater at birth was 2.0 percent or less.

## *ICSI*

Intracytoplasmic sperm injection (ICSI), or single sperm injection, is used in more than 60 percent of IVF cycles in the United States. Using

### ICSI AND FUTURE FERTILITY

Doctors argue that a version of IVF treatment that places individual sperm into eggs may be being overused and the consequence may be infertility of offspring. In normal IVF the sperm and egg are placed into a petri dish and the sperm breaks into and fertilizes the egg on its own, but in intracytoplasmic sperm injection (ICSI) it is the doctors who inject the sperm into the egg. A side effect of ICSI is that abnormal sperm may be injected into the egg which would otherwise be filtered out by the natural process of fertilization. Regardless of this consequence many British clinics have opted to use ICSI over IVF since its introduction in 1992; today two-thirds of fertility treatments in Europe are ICSI. Doctors claim that ICSI may have an increased risk of birth defects among offspring so it is better to use IVF. While ICSI may continue to be used at a high rate, it is necessary that patients are aware of possible risks to using ICSI.

Sources: Richard Alleyne, "IVF Technique a Fertility Threat to Next Generation," *The Telegraph,* Feb. 22, 2010, telegraph.co.uk.
Lois Rogers, "Test-tube Boys May Inherit Fertility Problems," *Times Online,* Feb. 7, 2010, Timesonline.co.uk.

a microscope and micromanipulation, the egg is held in place, and a small opening is made in it. Then a single sperm is injected into the egg. This process requires one egg and one motile sperm, as well as much technological expertise, and adds some risk as well as another expense ($1,000–$1,500)[25] to the process of IVF.

Prior to the advent of ICSI, natural processes prevented most abnormal sperm from entering the egg. The question of whether birth defects increase due to defective sperm being able to penetrate the egg has been only partially answered. A recent follow-up study of IVF pregnancies noted an increased risk of stillbirth for babies conceived through IVF/ICSI; this is in addition to the risk of preterm delivery for IVF babies.[26]

Some studies have noted an increase in certain male genitourinary system malformations, such as hypospadias, in boys born through ICSI.[27] Two syndromes, both rare, seem to have an increased incidence in IVF/ICSI. These are Angelman syndrome[28] and Beckwith-Wiedemann syndrome;[29] although they are increased in IVF/ICSI, their incidence is still low. Since it is not possible to look inside the sperm and see if it contains defective genetic material, this will be a risk for couples considering this technique. Additionally, the oldest children born through ICSI are now reaching reproductive age, so the effect of ICSI on male fertility in the next generation is yet to be seen.

## In Conclusion

GIFT, ZIFT, and IVF can all be used by couples without raising ethical concerns, as long as they are used within certain guidelines informed by the belief that personhood begins at conception. The couples who use these procedures should be committed to giving every embryo created in the lab an opportunity for implantation and development, so that no embryos are discarded or destroyed. Further, the number of embryos transferred should be no greater than the number of children the couple is willing to bear and rear, and no more than the woman can safely carry. Though this can increase the financial risk to couples in these procedures, it minimizes the moral risk of a callous disregard for unborn personhood.

Although these procedures are generally morally acceptable with the above guidelines, that does not mean that every time a couple uses one of them, they are exempt from doing so unethically. These procedures are very expensive, and are no guarantee of a live birth. Couples should be careful to be good stewards of their financial resources, and be willing to set limits on how far they will go in order to have a child through technological assistance. We would counsel couples to think about those limits prior to beginning infertility treatments. We would further urge couples to continue to exercise trust in a sovereign and trustworthy God. These technologies are the result of His common grace to human beings, but must be utilized within moral limits in order to safeguard the dignity of unborn human persons.

*Though surrogacy is an ancient remedy for infertility, what makes it novel today is the legal context in which it occurs.*

# CHAPTER SEVEN

# Surrogate Motherhood

When did it begin?

Perhaps it was the loneliness, the whispers of other women around her; the pitying looks as other women's bellies grew larger, and hers didn't. The meals for two, plus their servants and guests, continue d, with no child of their own to share their table. Her incredible beauty could not compensate for her sadness.

Then the idea came. She thought it brilliant, and told her husband; he agreed. He would try to impregnate her maid. If it worked, it would be like having a child of their own running around their home.

Well, it worked all right, but it didn't work out at all the way she thought it would. Hagar's son was not the son Sarah had expected to obtain. Yes, he was the son of her husband, but also the son of another woman. More than a decade passed before she herself became pregnant. Sarah gave birth to Isaac. After he had been weaned, she and Abraham hosted a party. She looked up to see Ishmael, about fourteen years of age, taunting her own son. She could not—she would not—countenance the son of a slave being the heir to Abraham's estate. So he—this child whom she had encouraged her husband to conceive—and Hagar, his mother, were sent away from Sarah and Abraham, who then reared Isaac as their only child.

Such is the story of the first recorded surrogate.

## A Controversial Gift of Life

From this inauspicious beginning, surrogate motherhood has remained a controversial, if increasingly common, reproductive technology. In many cases, the surrogate bears the child for the contracting couple, willingly gives up the child she has borne to the couple, and accepts her role with moderate to no difficulty.

In those cases, the contracting couple views the surrogate with extreme gratitude for helping their dream of having a child come true. The surrogate also feels a great deal of satisfaction, since she has in effect given a "gift of life" to a previously infertile couple.

But in some well-publicized cases, the surrogate has had a different experience. She has found that she wants to keep the child she has borne and fights for custody. What began as a harmonious relationship between the couple and the surrogate ends with numerous doubts about the wisdom of using this type of reproductive arrangement.

Though surrogacy is an ancient remedy for infertility, what makes surrogacy novel today is the *legal* context in which reproduction now occurs. The presence of lawyers, detailed contracts, and even the idea of legal representation for the yet to be born child are the new elements in the previously very private area of procreation.

### Genetic Surrogacy

There are a wide variety of surrogacy arrangements that are possible today. The simplest form of surrogacy is what is called *genetic surrogacy* (or traditional surrogacy), in which the surrogate contributes both her egg and womb to the couple who contracts her services. The surrogate is genetically related to the child she is carrying since through her egg, she supplies half of the child's DNA.

Typically, she becomes pregnant by intrauterine insemination with sperm from the man in the contracting couple, carries the child to term, gives birth, and turns over custody to the contracting couple. Couples who cannot conceive a child because of the inability of the woman to produce eggs might consider a genetic surrogate, though if the lack of egg production is the only problem and the woman can otherwise carry a pregnancy, the couple may opt for an egg donor alone (in which case the husband's sperm would be used in IVF and the embryos would be implanted in the womb of his wife, who would carry the child to term, give birth, and assume the role of social mother of the child).

Genetic surrogacy was very popular in the early days of surrogacy when both IVF and egg harvesting were in their infancy. Its popularity has waned dramatically for heterosexual couples, given that both egg donation and IVF have become more routine practices. In addition, in many states, genetic surrogates have rights to their child, bringing in potential legal complications should a disagreement about custody of the child arise.

However, gay men, who can provide the sperm for intrauterine insemination, need genetic surrogates in order to have children. They have become some of the primary customers for genetic surrogacy.

### Gestational Surrogacy

In other cases, the infertile woman may be able to produce eggs but cannot carry a pregnancy to term. A *gestational surrogate* may be recruited. This is a more complicated and more expensive case, since in

## NEW LAW AFFECTS GAY MEN AND SURROGACY

On April 6, 2010, an addition to the 2008 Human Fertilisation and Embryology Act (UK) made it legal for two men to be named the parents of a child born through surrogacy. Legislators hope the addition will give same-sex and unmarried couples the ability to use surrogacy as a means to securing legal parenthood. Prior to this new law, legislation only permitted heterosexual, married couples to obtain a parental order to have a birth certificate with both parents' names on it. The surrogate mother had to be on the birth certificate, and if she was married, her husband's name also had to be on the birth certificate. Since lesbian and unmarried couples often have other alternatives to surrogacy, this law is especially beneficial for same-sex couples to become parents.

Source: Robin McKie, "New Surrogacy Law Eases the Way for Gay Men to Become Legal Parents," *The Observer*, March 28, 2010, guardian.co.uk.

vitro fertilization is also required.

The surrogate has no genetic tie to the child she is carrying. In these cases, the woman has her eggs harvested through the same procedure that is used for IVF. Then the eggs are fertilized with her husband's sperm, and the resulting embryos transferred to implant in a surrogate's womb. She carries the pregnancy to term, gives birth, and then hands over custody of the child/children to the contracting couple.

A gestational surrogate may be involved with use of donor gametes. That is to say, donor sperm and egg(s) are used in IVF, and the resulting embryo(s) gestated by the surrogate. The two parents who are genetically unrelated to the child (the ones who hired the surrogate and arranged for the donor gametes) rear the child. In gestational surrogacy, then, as many as five separate people can contribute to the conception, birth, and upbringing of a single child.

In one of the most bizarre surrogacy cases on record, a California couple, John and Luanne Buzzanca, created a child using donor eggs and sperm. They hired a surrogate mother to have the in vitro–created embryo implanted and to carry the child. The Buzzancas intended to raise the child.

Two weeks after the Buzzancas signed a contract with the surrogate, they separated and John filed for divorce one month prior to the child's birth, thus leaving the little girl in temporary legal limbo. It was finally resolved with the Buzzancas taking responsibility for the child—Luanne reared her and John contributed child support.[1]

### Commercial and Altruistic Surrogacy

When the surrogate is paid a fee for the entire process, it is called *commercial surrogacy*. Most surrogates are paid for what they do, usually thousands of dollars in addition to all medical expenses; sometimes even lost wages due to the pregnancy are reimbursed. But once in a while, a family member or close friend offers to carry a child for an infertile woman simply out of a desire to give the "gift of life." When this happens, it is called *altruistic surrogacy*. Both genetic and gestational surrogacy can be done commercially or altruistically.

The following two precedent-setting cases illustrate the myriad of complexities that can occur in a surrogate parenting arrangement.

### The Baby M Case[2]

In the soap-opera drama of the first well-publicized surrogacy case, which took place in 1986 and eventually became a television movie, William Stern had a special interest in fathering a child to whom he was genetically related. He was the only living member of his bloodline; most of his relatives had been killed during the Holocaust. His wife, Elizabeth, thought she had a mild case of multiple sclerosis and she believed that the health risk of pregnancy was significant.

The Infertility Center of New York matched the Sterns with Mary Beth Whitehead, a woman of moderate means with two children already. She agreed to be inseminated with Stern's sperm (thus making it a case of genetic surrogacy), and surrender custody of the child upon birth for a $10,000 fee and all associated medical expenses. If she miscarried prior to the fifth month, she would receive no fee, but if miscarriage came after the fifth month or if the child was stillborn, she would receive $1,000.

After the child was born, Whitehead sued for custody after regretting her decision to give up the child to the Sterns. The Sterns allowed her to take the child for a week, after which time she fled the area with the child. The police later recovered the child in Florida, and by force returned her to the Sterns.

In a decision handed down in March 1987, the New Jersey Superior Court ruled that the surrogacy contract between the Sterns and Whitehead was valid. Judge Harvey Sorkow ruled that Whitehead had not been coerced into signing the contract and therefore it should be enforced.

Using the analogy between a sperm donation and a woman "renting her womb," he ruled that a woman had the right to sell her reproductive capacities. Thus Whitehead breached a valid contract when she refused to surrender the child and give up custody.

Even though the contract was upheld, a custody hearing was held since the best interests of the child was the primary concern. The judge ruled that custody should be given to the Sterns since they would be able to provide a more stable home for the child.

Upon appeal to the New Jersey Supreme Court, the decision was reversed; William Stern was the baby's legal father and Mary Beth Whitehead rather than Elizabeth Stern was her *legal* mother. However, the final custody outcome remained the same—the baby would go to the Sterns. Judge Robert Wilentz, writing for a unanimous Court, ruled that surrogacy contracts violated the state laws that prohibit the transfer of money for adoptions. Surrogacy was, in effect, baby-selling, and there are some things—namely, human life—that cannot be bought or sold. They cited as evidence the way the fee was paid to Whitehead. Significantly less money was to be paid Whitehead if the baby was miscarried or stillborn. Clearly the Sterns were paying for a child and full parental rights, not just rental of her womb.

The Court also cited New Jersey laws that held the fundamental rights of genetic parents to participate in raising their children. Since Mary Beth Whitehead was not an unfit mother and had not abandoned her child, there was no good reason to deny her the right of association. In addition, the contract violated laws that stipulated a time period for an adoptive mother to change her mind prior to irrevocably giving up her child. Further, the contract violated established New Jersey public policy on custody that gave the natural parents the right to determine who would raise the child. However, precedent dictated that that decision cannot be made prior to the child's birth.

The adoption of the child by Elizabeth Stern (facilitated by Judge Sorkow immediately after his lower court decision) was voided and Whitehead was to get visitation rights to be decided by a lower court. She did not receive custody since the justices held that the child's best interests would be served by custody of the Sterns. Even though Mary Beth announced a pregnancy by another man shortly thereafter and separated from her husband, visitation rights were not terminated.

### *Calvert v. Johnson*[3]

In October 1990, another precedent-setting case was decided. In Orange County, California, Mark and Crispina Calvert hired Anna Johnson to be the surrogate mother for their child. This case was different from Baby M in that the surrogate had no genetic relationship to the child. She agreed to carry a pregnancy for the Calverts, for $10,000 plus all medical expenses.

Toward the beginning of the seventh month, Johnson started having second thoughts about giving up the child she was bearing. A month prior to the child's birth, Johnson sued for custody. When the child was born in mid-September, temporary custody was awarded to the Calverts with daily visitation allowed to Johnson. These were later reduced to twice weekly until the final custody hearing.

Orange County Superior Court Judge Richard Parslow ruled that the surrogacy contract was valid, and not inherently exploitive. Since Anna Johnson had no genetic stake in the child, she had no parental rights. Thus exclusive custody of the child was given to the Calverts and no visitation allowed.

The judge ruled that the genetic connection took precedence over the fact that Johnson actually gave birth to the child, and that best interests of the child would be served by custody of the Calverts in any case.

Some testimony was given that undermined Johnson's fitness as a mother. Her roommate testified to the neglect of her current child; and the fact that she was a single mother with minimal financial resources who had difficulty holding down a job contributed to the decision to award custody to the Calverts. In addition, the sincerity of her bond to the child was questioned since she didn't mention until the seventh month of the pregnancy that she was forming ties to the baby; and these statements contradicted numerous earlier statements she had made to the Calverts as she was carrying their child.

### *Lessons to Heed*

In both of these cases, an infertile couple hired a surrogate through an intermediary agency to bear a child for them, with what they considered a valid contract governing the procedure. All medical expenses related to the pregnancy were paid by the contracting couple, and the surrogate was to receive a fee of $10,000 for specific performance of the contract.

In each case the surrogate changed her mind and sued to retain parental rights to the child she had borne, and the judges, in deciding each respective case, were setting new precedents, since neither had any significant legal precedent upon which they could base their decision. In New Jersey, Baby M was the first surrogacy case to receive broad legal and public attention. But in California, the precedent set in New Jersey was not that helpful since the relation of the surrogate to the child was different. What made this case more difficult is that the law presumes that the birth mother is the legal mother, based on the assumption that genetics and gestation go together. The end result of the two cases was the same, in that the contracting couple was given permanent custody of the child, though the way in which the surrogacy contract was viewed was quite different. The court found in each case that the best interests of the child would be served by living with the contracting couple.

There were some significant differences between the two cases, however. The principal difference was the place of genetic relationship between the surrogate and the child. Whitehead was the genetic mother, having supplied the egg, whereas Johnson was the gestational mother, with no genetic link to the child. Thus the view of the surrogacy contract was different. In New Jersey, the judge ruled that the contract was void because it required Whitehead to give up a fundamental right to parent. But in California, the judge ruled that the contract was valid and since there was no genetic link between the surrogate and the child, there were no parental rights to be considered.

Johnson, therefore, had no choice but to give the child to the people the judge considered to be the parents. Genetics made all the difference in the custody award in the Calvert case and in voiding the New Jersey contract. Though the view of the contract was quite different, each child ended up with the contracting couple. Whitehead was granted liberal visitation rights and Johnson was granted none—a reflection of the Court's high view of a parent's genetic contribution to children.

In addition, the fitness of the surrogate as a mother was considered differently by the courts. Though Whitehead came in for harsh criticism in the lower court, the New Jersey Supreme Court ruled that she was indeed fit as a mother and that the lower court had been unfairly biased against her. In Orange County, the judge raised significant questions about Johnson's fitness as a mother based on the testimony of her roommate, her status as a single parent, and her employment history.

**WASHINGTON MAKES SURROGACY LEGAL**

House Bill 2793 in Washington was created to clarify and expand the parenting rights and responsibilities of domestic partners and other couples. The bill is twofold: it amends the Uniform Parentage Act (UPA); and sets standards for gestational surrogacy contracts. The amendments made to the UPA include the qualification that terms such as *spouse, marriage, husband*, and *wife* must allow for an interpretation that applies equally to domestic partnerships and marital relationships, and when necessary, gender-specific terms must be interpreted as gender neutral. Also, the bill established standards and requirements of gestational surrogacy for both intended parents and surrogate mothers, including the need to have a proper gestational surrogacy contract between both parties.

## Moral Assessment of Surrogate Motherhood

Every surrogacy arrangement involves a third party who is central to bringing a child into the world. In view of the biblical skepticism concerning third party contributors in general, which we discussed in chapter 2, we would suggest that surrogacy is outside the prima facie norm of procreation taking place within the sacred context of marriage.

Bringing a surrogate into the process of procreation is an intrusion to the marital bond, from which procreation should occur. All forms of surrogacy involve this problematic element, whether they are genetic or gestational, or whether they are done for a profit or altruistically. Thus in terms of the general theological assessment of surrogacy, we find it difficult to see any grounds on which most surrogacy arrangements could go forward without violating God's original design for procreation.

This position is similar to the position we outlined in chapter 5 when it involved sperm and egg donors. To be consistent, we are not arguing that all surrogacy is necessarily sin, and we have a small handful of scenarios in which we hold that surrogacy would be acceptable. We do hold that most surrogacy arrangements run contrary to the trajectory of Scripture, which is skeptical of procreative arrangements that are outside the context of marriage, since they include a third party contributor who is arguably more involved than an anonymous sperm or egg donor.

However, there are other moral considerations that are relevant to surrogacy, which present additional causes for concern. Some of these are applicable to all types of surrogacy arrangements, and others are unique to one form of surrogacy (genetic or gestational), or to commercial surrogacy, where money beyond reasonable expenses is changing hands. We realize that there is considerable debate over a key issue in surrogacy—that is, the definition of the mother, especially in gestational surrogacy situations.

It is widely held both morally and in the law that a *genetic/traditional surrogate*—who contributes the egg, carries the pregnancy, and gives birth to the child—*is the mother, with full maternal rights to her child*. But gestational surrogacy, in which the surrogate has no genetic relationship to the child she bears, is a more complicated scenario. If we conclude that there is a major difference between the two types of surrogacy arrangements, then the moral discussion will be somewhat different. But if we conclude that genetic and gestational surrogates are similarly situated, then the same objections to genetic surrogacy will also apply to gestational surrogacy. We'll begin with some of the moral concerns with genetic, commercial surrogacy.

## *Surrogacy Involves the Purchase and Sale of Children*

Certainly the most serious objection to commercial surrogacy is that it reduces children to objects of barter by putting a price on them. Of course, if the surrogacy arrangement is done without a fee paid to the surrogate, then the charge of surrogacy being the sale of children does not hold. But since most surrogacy contracts do involve a fee to the surrogate beyond expenses, the charge of baby-selling is difficult to avoid.

This is most clear in the case of the genetic surrogate, who is clearly the mother, when she turns over custody of her child and signs away her maternal rights, in exchange for a cash payment. If the parties involved in this type of surrogacy arrangement were attempting an adoption, and the adoptive parents were paying the birth mother a five-figure fee beyond her expenses, they would be in violation of the law—since adoption law prohibits paying birth mothers to give up their children for adoption, precisely because it constitutes the purchase and sale of children.

Of course, whether or not gestational surrogacy also involves baby-selling depends on the definition of motherhood in surrogacy arrangements. If the gestational surrogate is also the mother, then gestational surrogacy also constitutes baby-selling, and the argument in this section applies to that form of surrogacy too. But if the gestational surrogate is not the mother, then the charge of baby-selling would not apply, since the surrogate would not be receiving the fee in exchange for turning over rights to her child, but rather for something like "pregnancy services rendered."

In fact, we would suggest that most of the arguments in favor of surrogacy are attempts to avoid or minimize this problem. Opponents of surrogacy insist that any attempt to deny or minimize the charge of baby-selling fails, and thus surrogacy involves the sale of children. This violates the thirteenth amendment that outlawed slavery because it constituted the sale of human beings. It violates commonly and widely held moral principles that safeguard human rights and the dignity of human persons, namely, that human beings are made in God's image and are His unique creations. Persons are not fundamentally things that can be purchased and sold for a price.

The fact that proponents of surrogacy try so hard to get around the charge of baby-selling indicates their acceptance of these moral principles as well. The debate is not whether human beings should be bought and sold. Rather it is over whether commercial surrogacy constitutes such a sale of children. If it does, most would agree that the case against this form of surrogacy is quite strong. As the New Jersey Supreme Court put it in the Baby M case, "There are, in a civilized society, some things that money cannot buy. . . . There are values . . . that society deems more important than granting to wealth whatever it can buy, be it labor, love or life."[4]

The sale of children, which normally results from a surrogacy transaction (the only exception being cases of altruistic surrogacy), is inherently problematic, irrespective of the other good consequences that the arrangement produces, in the same way that slavery is inherently troubling, because human beings are not objects for sale.

Surrogacy proponents are sensitive to the charge that paying a surrogate a large amount of money for bearing a child for another couple is baby-selling. Therefore, the argument is that the fee only pays for gestational services rendered, and is not the sale of a child. Proponents insist that it is only fair for a woman to be compensated for her time, risk, and sacrifice that pregnancy entails. People have a right to be compensated appropriately for services rendered. Just as it is legitimate to pay surrogate child-rearers in a day care setting, proponents insist that it should be legitimate to pay surrogate child-bearers.

This argument fails to take into account that the fee is for much more than childbirth services rendered. The service provided in bearing the child is clearly not the intended end product of the arrangement. What really counts in a surrogacy arrangement is not only the successful birth of the child but also the transfer of parental rights from the surrogate to the infertile wife. She must adopt the child and receive custody in order for the deal to be done.

In genetic surrogacy cases, in which the surrogate supplies both the egg and the womb, she is the legal mother of the child. Under the law, should she so desire, she may keep the child and share custody with the natural father. Thus, for any surrogacy arrangement to be completed, she must turn over her parental rights to the child. Opponents of surrogacy insist that the fee also pays for this transfer of parental rights, and is thus baby-selling.

For example, in the well-known Baby M case, only in the event of the surrogate's delivering a healthy baby to the contracting couple and turning over parental rights, would she be paid the full $10,000 fee. If she miscarried prior to the fifth month of pregnancy, she would receive nothing. If she miscarried after the fifth month or gave birth to a stillborn child, she would receive only $1,000. The contract was clearly oriented to the delivery of the end product, not the gestational process.

To be consistent, if the fee paid to the surrogate is only for gestational services rendered, the surrogate would be paid the same amount whether or not she turned over the child to the contracting couple. If the fee only pays for childbirth services, it is hard to see how a couple could take the surrogate to court to get the child, since the surrogate would have fulfilled her part of the contract once the child was born. In addition, if she miscarried at some point in the pregnancy, her fee should be prorated over the number of months that she performed a gestational service. Advocates of surrogacy insist that this would make surrogacy much too risky for the contracting couple.

In our view, a successful surrogacy depends on the delivery of the product—the child—thus the actual practice of surrogacy suggests that it is far more than simply a "fee for service" arrangement.

Proponents of surrogacy will respond that the natural father cannot buy back what is already his, and thus surrogacy cannot be babyselling. But the child is not *all* his. At best, he can only claim the equivalent of joint tenancy in a piece of property, in which he "buys out" his partner, the surrogate, and thus is still baby-selling.[5]

Some proponents of surrogacy will admit that children are being sold, but that the circumstances are so different from black market adoptions that it does no harm to exchange parental rights for money. The laws that prevent payment to birth mothers were designed to prevent black market adoptions, in which birth mothers were exploited based on their financial need and in which the well-being of the children was not considered the highest priority.

Surrogacy is a completely different situation. Here the natural father is also the adopting father, and surrogacy results from a planned and wanted pregnancy as opposed to an unwanted pregnancy. Thus the child is not going to a stranger but to a genetic relative, and the surrogate is not coerced into making a decision she will later regret.

Opponents of surrogacy respond that the differences between black market adoptions and surrogacy are understated. For example, there is little screening of the contracting couple done in order to ensure that they are fit parents and that the best interests of the child are being maintained. In addition, the element of coercion is not entirely absent from a surrogacy arrangement since it is quite possible that the surrogate could end up being coerced by the contract into giving up a child that she may realize she wants to keep. Further, given the desperation of the contracting couple to have a child, since they usually do not resort to surrogacy until all other means have been exhausted, they are open to exploitation by the surrogacy brokers. Thus to say that the environment surrounding surrogacy is free from coercion is not accurate.

Even if the child is treated well and the arrangement comes off without coercion, the problem of baby-selling remains. Likewise, during the antebellum years in our nation, there were cases in which slaves were treated well and considered to be family members, but the fact remained that they had been bought and sold and had become objects of barter. The circumstances in which such barter takes place is irrelevant according to opponents of surrogacy.

## Surrogacy Involves Potential for Exploitation of the Surrogate

Most agree about the potential for commercial surrogacy to be exploitative, applicable to both genetic and gestational surrogates. This is not to say that altruistic surrogacy cannot ever be exploitive, for not all exploitation is financially based. Without money changing hands, altruistic surrogacy seems less likely to be exploitative.

In commercial surrogacy, the combination of desperate infertile couples, low-income surrogates, and profit-minded surrogacy brokers raises the prospect that the entire commercial enterprise can be exploitative. With the trend toward outsourcing surrogacy to some of the most impoverished parts of the world, concern about exploitation is growing.[6]

For some of the surrogates from the developing world, the fee paid to them is sometimes the equivalent of many months of wages, if not a full year or more. It offers them the opportunity to purchase a home, pay off debts, or just survive a bit more comfortably. Of course, the existence of the fee alone should not be considered exploitation. Without being exploitative, money often functions as an inducement

## OUTSOURCING SURROGACY

In March 2008 the Rajiv Gandhi International airport opened in Hyderabad, India. With the opening of the airport came an increase of clientele to mid-sized health centers that offer infertility treatment and surrogacy. Since commercial surrogacy was legalized in India in 2002, people from around the globe have been traveling to India to find surrogate mothers. In the past two years, doctors at Hyderabad have seen the number of couples seeking surrogate mothers double. India and the United States are two countries that have legalized surrogacy, and many couples opt for finding surrogate mothers in India over the United States because it is safe, hassle-free, and available at a more reasonable price than in the United States. Also, agencies around the world are sending people to India for surrogacy. However, there are two concerns with the rise of surrogacy in India: it may be hard to find surrogate mothers since many parts of India are still very conservative, and some fear the trend of surrogacy is turning Indian women into baby factories.

Sources: Bella Jaisinghani, "Maid-to-order Surrogate Mums," *The Times of India*, April 11, 2010, timesofIndia.indiatimes.com.
"Swanky Airport Puts Hyderabad on World's Surrogacy Map," *The Times of India*, Feb. 20, 2010, timesofindia.indiatimes.com.
"Commercial Surrogacy a Booming Industry Now," *Gulf Times*, March 10, 2010, Gulf-times.com.

to do many things that people would not normally undertake.

However, this does not mean that the potential for exploitation should not be taken seriously. It is not difficult to imagine that one day surrogacy could be entirely outsourced in order to hold down costs and to maximize the profit of the brokers. Some are even suggesting that those with financial need actually make the best candidates for surrogates since they are the least inclined to keep the child produced by the arrangement.[7]

Surrogacy is a part of what is becoming known as "reproductive tourism," in which those with money and a demand for surrogacy travel to hub destinations where the surrogacy industry is developing. Some places in the developing world, such as in India, openly advertise themselves as the lowest cost options for couples seeking surrogates. Krittivas Mukherjee reported on the situation in 2007:

> "In the U.S. a childless couple would have to spend anything up to $50,000," Gautam Allahbadia, a fertility specialist who helped a Singaporean couple obtain a child through an Indian surrogate last year, told Reuters.
>
> "In India, it's done for $10,000–$12,000."
>
> Fertility clinics usually charge $2,000–$3,000 for the procedure while a surrogate is paid anything between $3,000 and $6,000, a fortune in a country with an annual per capita income of around $500.[8]

The advantage to using these women is that it dramatically reduces the cost of doing the surrogacy business. One surrogacy broker stated that the surrogates from these countries would only receive the basic necessities and travel expenses for their services, and in many cases would not even have to travel at all. Revealing a strong bias toward exploitation of the surrogates, he stated, "Often they [the potential surrogates] are looking for a survival situation—something to do to pay for the rent and food. They come from underdeveloped countries where food is a serious issue." But he also added that they make good candidates for surrogacy when he stated, "They know how to take care of children . . . it's obviously a perfect match."[9]

He further speculates that perhaps one-tenth of the normal fee could be paid these women and it would not even matter if they had some other health problems, as long as they had an adequate diet and no problems that would affect the developing child.[10] It is not difficult to see the potential for crass exploitation of poor women in desperate circumstances.

## Surrogacy Violates the Right of Mothers to Associate with Their Children

Another serious problem with commercial surrogacy might also apply to altruistic surrogacy. In most surrogacy contracts, whether for a fee or not, the surrogate agrees to relinquish any parental rights to the child she is carrying to the couple who contracted her services. In the Baby M case, the police actually had to break into a home to return the baby to the contracting couple.[11] A surrogacy contract forces a woman to give up the child she has borne to the couple who has paid her to do so. Should she have second thoughts and desire to keep the child, under the contract she would be forced to give up her child.

Of course, whether or not surrogacy violates this right depends on the definition of the mother in these arrangements. In cases of genetic surrogacy, in which the surrogate provides both the genetic material and the womb, she is clearly the mother of the child. To force her to give up her child under the terms of a surrogacy contract violates her fundamental right to associate with and rear her child.[12] This does not mean, however, that she has exclusive right to the child. That must be shared with the natural father, similar to a custody arrangement in a divorce proceeding. But the right of one parent (the natural father) to associate with his child should not be enforced at the expense of the right of the other (the surrogate).

In cases of gestational surrogacy, if the surrogate is the mother, then the same objection would hold. But if the gestational surrogate

## GUIDELINES FOR SURROGACY FOR CLINICS IN INDIA

**3.5.3** The ART clinic must not be a party to any commercial element in donor programmes or in gestational surrogacy.

**3.5.4** A surrogate mother carrying a child biologically unrelated to her must register as a patient in her own name. While registering she must mention that she is a surrogate mother and provide all the necessary information about the genetic parents such as names, addresses, etc. She must not use/register in the name of the person for whom she is carrying the child, as this would pose legal issues, particularly in the untoward event of maternal death (in whose names will the hospital certify this death?). The birth certificate shall be in the name of the genetic parents. The clinic, however, must also provide a certificate to the genetic parents giving the name and address of the surrogate mother. All the expenses of the surrogate mother during the period of pregnancy and post-natal care relating to pregnancy should be borne by the couple seeking surrogacy. The surrogate mother would also be entitled to a monetary compensation from the couple for agreeing to act as a surrogate; the exact value of this compensation should be decided by discussion between the couple and the proposed surrogate mother. An oocyte donor can not act as a surrogate mother for the couple to whom the ooctye is being donated.

Source: *Guidelines for ART Clinics in India*, chapter 3, http://icmr.nic.in/art/art_clinics.htm.

is not invested with maternal rights, then she is not giving up her child, and no fundamental right of association is violated.

As a result of this fundamental right of a mother to bond and have a relationship with her child, even if one allows a fee to be paid to the genetic surrogate, it's problematic to have their agreement enforced if the surrogate wants to keep the child. Any agreement that requires a woman prior to birth to agree to give up the child she bears is not considered a valid contract.

This is similar to the way that most states deal with adoptions. Any agreement prior to birth to give up a birth mother's child is not binding and can be revoked if the birth mother changes her mind and wants to keep the child. Some object to this and say that the surrogate is an adult and "a deal's a deal." But in civilized societies, some deals are not a deal—they are inherently invalid.

Say, for example, that my coauthor Dr. Riley and I have a difference about some feature of this book—one about which we both feel very strongly. Suppose that we decide that we'll settle our differences the old-fashioned way, with a duel—pistols at twenty paces. We both sign a contract and specify a date and time for our duel. If one of us backs out of the deal, the other could not go to court to enforce our contract. In fact, we'd both be laughed out of court, and justifiably so. The reason is that, even though we are both adults and "a deal's a deal," the contract to engage in a duel is inherently invalid and unenforceable since keeping it would result in a death.

Similarly, the courts have said that a woman cannot be forced by contract to give up her children, unless she is unfit. This was one of the most egregious problems with slavery—that it forcibly took children away from their mothers against their will.

Upholding this right of women to associate with their children and thereby allowing the surrogate to keep the child if she so desires substantially increases the risk of surrogacy to the contracting couple. They might go through the entire process and end up with shared custody of a child that they initially thought was to be all theirs. To many people, that doesn't seem fair, unless the rights of the surrogate are clearly disclosed prior to signing the agreement. However, we would suggest that it is more unfair to take a child away from his or her mother on the basis of a contract.

### Surrogacy Involves Detachment from the Child In Utero

One of the most serious objections to surrogacy applies to all types of surrogacy arrangements. In screening women to select the most ideal surrogates, one looks for the woman's ability to give up the child she is carrying without second thoughts. Normally, the less attached the woman is to the child, the easier it is to complete the arrangement.

But this is hardly an ideal setting for a pregnancy. Surrogacy sanctions female detachment from the child in the womb, a situation that in any other pregnancy one would never want. This detachment is something that would be strongly discouraged in a traditional pregnancy, yet is strongly encouraged in surrogacy. Thus surrogacy actually turns a vice, the ability to detach from the child in utero, into a virtue. A case in point is Jill Hawkins, a single British woman who was interviewed during her eighth surrogate pregnancy:

> Miss Hawkins, from Brighton, said: "It's a new experience this time because they are not my biological children. I feel different. I feel there's not so much pressure on me because it's not my genes. I'm just providing the womb for the baby to grow in."[13]

Another example of this expectation on the surrogate comes from a gay British couple: Jonathan, who with his partner, Colin, paid a total of $150,000 for expenses, including a California surrogate to have a baby for them. They put it this way:

> We had our own child and had a great team to help us. All we did was rent a woman to carry her. We paid for the services of an embryologist and an incubator who walks and makes good babies—but we didn't buy a baby. She's my daughter biologically, and she's our baby.[14]

Should surrogacy be widely practiced, bioethicist Daniel Callahan of the Hastings Center describes what one of the results would be. He states, "We will be forced to cultivate the services of women with the hardly desirable trait of being willing to gestate and then give up their own children, especially if paid enough to do so. . . .There would still be the need to find women with the capacity to dissociate and distance themselves from their own child. This is not a psychological trait we should want to foster, even in the name of altruism."[15]

Law professor Katharine Bartlett puts it this way in expressing this concern: "[Surrogacy] presupposes that the biological mother-child bond is easily severed, that pregnancy and childbirth is a process that does not necessarily entail enduring human emotion and permanent connectedness, that women can have children and give them up if the price is right, and that women who make such agreements and change their minds are acting improperly, even pathologically."[16]

These concerns would exist whether or not the surrogate is being paid, and whether or not she is the recognized mother of the child. In fact, it may be more of a concern in cases of gestational surrogacy, since the surrogate has no genetic connection to the child and may find it easier to detach herself emotionally from the child she is carrying.

## Defining Motherhood in Surrogacy

In the cases of genetic surrogacy, the definition of motherhood is straightforward and not particularly controversial. The Baby M decision set the precedent for how cases of genetic surrogacy would be handled if the surrogate desires to keep the child. The only dissenting voice in this area comes from those who hold that the *intention to parent*, expressed in the surrogacy contract, should be that which ultimately determines who is the mother in these arrangements.[17] It should be noted that the American College of Obstetricians and Gynecologists does not address the issue of "Who's the mommy?"; rather, ACOG simply acknowledges the possibilities in its ethics committee's opinion on surrogate motherhood:

> The different types of relationships that are possible—genetic (either, both, or neither intended parent), gestational (the surrogate mother), and social or rearing (the intended parents)— give rise to both conceptual challenges regarding the nature of parenthood and legal problems as to who should be considered the parents responsible for the child.[18]

The most controversial of all the surrogacy scenarios is gestational surrogacy, in which the surrogate has no genetic relationship to the child she is carrying. It even necessitates clarification of the term "biological mother," since that encompasses both the genetic and gestational elements, which can now be separated in surrogacy. We will briefly look at the case for each: gestation, genetics, and intention as the determinants of motherhood.

### Gestation Determines Motherhood

The view that gestation determines motherhood reflects the traditional view of parental rights. In this view the woman who gives birth to the child is conclusively presumed to be the mother of the child, with full, uncontested maternal rights.

This position reflects the view of the Warnock Report in England, which looked ahead to anticipate gestational surrogacy, although surrogacy at that time was not permitted in the UK. As in cases where the egg or embryo is donated, the "donation should be treated as absolute," and the donors have no inherent parental rights to the child. Thus the woman giving birth is regarded as the mother of the child.[19]

## A SURROGATE MOTHER GOES TO COURT

In New Jersey a judge ruled that a gestational surrogate mother of twins who was not the biological mother was the legal mother and could pursue custody of the children. Angelina Robinson agreed to be a surrogate mother for her brother, Donald Robinson Hollingsworth, and his partner, Sean Hollingsworth. An anonymous donor's eggs and Sean Hollingsworth's sperm were implanted in Angelina's womb. The twins were born and handed over to the Hollingsworths in October 2006. In March 2007 Ms. Robinson took her brother and his partner to court, arguing that they had coerced her into being a surrogate. If the ruling is upheld, the rights of gestational surrogacy may be expanded. As of now, states in the United States have not standardized surrogacy laws in the country. Professor Kindregan at Suffolk University Law School is working to enact standard surrogacy laws across the U.S. and help avoid future problems for couples who use surrogacy.

Source: Stephanie Saul, "New Jersey Judge Calls Surrogate Legal Mother of Twins," *The New York Times*, Dec. 31, 2009, NYTimes.com.

The notion that gestation should determine motherhood is based principally on the contribution the gestational mother makes during pregnancy and birth. She is much more than a "human incubator," and makes a substantial contribution not only to the physical development of the child but to the child's emotional and psychological development as well.

As opposed to simply donating the egg, the gestational mother has built up what some call "sweat equity" in the child she is carrying.[20] The nine months' investment in the child and the labor, literally, involved in giving birth tilt the equation in favor of gestation. She clearly has made the greater investment in the child in terms of effort and time expended, and thus she should have a greater claim to motherhood.

At the end of the process of birth, the woman who bore the child will have contributed much more of herself than the egg donor in order to bring the child into the world. For a woman who knows what pregnancy and childbirth involve, the contribution of the egg donor might even seem trivial compared to the rigors and demands of the "around the clock" nature of pregnancy and birth.

Similar in importance to the investment and contribution of the gestational mother is the bonding that occurs between her and the child she is carrying. Though significant bonding can take place between any two individuals, the combination of biological investment and the resultant bonding weighs heavily in favor of gestation as the determinant of motherhood.[21] That is, the combination of biology and relationship that is inherent in gestation argues for motherhood being vested in the woman who bears the child.

In most pregnancies, this bond is a central part of the pregnant woman's self-concept, and though children do not normally entirely define a woman's life, they are surely integral to what defines her as a person. In most instances, the loss of this bond causes a great deal of grief when a pregnancy is lost. This is even the case in an adoption in which the birth mother realizes that giving up the child is in both the child's and her own best interests. One reason that many states have a period in which a birth mother can regain custody of her child prior to the adoption's becoming final is that they recognize the strength of this bond.

Most states do not hold an adoptive mother to a pre-birth consent to adoption, since she cannot know the strength of the bond she will feel with her child prior to birth, and thus cannot give genuinely informed consent. In the UK, birth mothers have six weeks during which to change their minds about adoption.[22] In cases in which the surrogate changes her mind and wants to keep the child, it is reasonable to see this bond as similarly important and self-defining.

Though one should be careful about affirming a "biology is destiny" concept of self for women, that is not to say that pregnancy, childbirth, and motherhood cannot be highly determinative of a woman's sense of self.

This sense of bonding is what makes pregnancy essentially a relationship, not only physiologically but emotionally. What makes a woman a mother is the unique relationship developed with the fetus in the nine months of pregnancy and the event of birth. Gestation creates motherhood because of the intense, intimate relationship that is created as a woman carries a developing child. Proponents of gestation as the definition of motherhood insist that egg donation and a five-figure fee paid to the surrogate do not compare with the bonding that has been established during pregnancy.

### Genetics Determines Motherhood

Particularly with the completion of the Human Genome Project, which mapped the human genetic code, there is little doubt about the importance of genetics in determining who a child becomes. The combination of genes is what gives each child his or her unique characteristics and traits, and those elements form a substantial part of each child's identity. Genetics is determinative of many things in an individual's life, from facial features to tendencies to acquire certain diseases.

The priority of genetics in determining motherhood is also suggested in cases in which the child bears a strong physical resemblance to one or both of the genetic contributors. Advocates of this position suggest that in cases like these, it is difficult to deny the very powerful influence of genetics, and even more difficult to deny parental rights to a child who looks like those who supplied the gametes. Thus if the contracting couple supplies both egg and sperm, genetics is a powerful criterion for assigning parental rights to them.[23]

In this situation, the surrogate mother is viewed as providing only the care and feeding of the child during the nine months of pregnancy. She may contribute relatively little to the physical features and traits of the child, assuming, of course, that she does not engage in behavior during the pregnancy that causes physical harm to the fetus. To take the idea of the "human incubator" a step further, if the embryo were implanted in another woman, the physical features would be the same. The child would look the same irrespective of who supplied the gestational environment. Because of this powerful connection between a child's genes and the important features that constitute his or her identity, it is argued that genetics should be the element that determines maternity.

This argument for genetics being the determining factor in motherhood is further illustrated by the strong desire of adopted children to reconnect with their natural parents. There is something significant about the genetic tie that frequently compels adopted children to go to great lengths simply to be reunited with their natural parents, even though they may have no intention of living with them. In fact, this often happens once a person becomes an adult, when there is no possibility of the parent providing anything for the child, as would be expected in the earlier years of the child's upbringing. The adult child simply has the desire to unite with the one whose genes he or she inherited.

Of course, there are occasions with other motives for seeking out a natural parent, for example, greed or anger, or to learn more about one's medical history. But often, there is no desire other than to make a connection with the person to whom one is genetically related, because those genes have made a substantial contribution to the identity of the individual. This is not to minimize the contribution of the social parent in developing the character of the child, if, for example, the child is adopted. Rather, it is to show the powerful genetic contribution in contrast to that made by the woman who simply carries the embryo to term and brings him/her into the world. This is further underscored by the growing number of children born from DI who are attempting to seek out previously anonymous sperm donors.[24] A further example of this is the Donor Sibling Registry, a database established to enable children born of donor gametes to connect with their biological parent and any stepsiblings.[25]

A final argument in favor of genetics as the maternal rights "trump card" is based on the concept that individuals own their own gametes.[26] The very notion of sperm and egg donation is premised on the idea that an individual owns his or her genetic material. It is a part of one's body just as is any other critical component. Whether it may be bought and sold is another issue, and it does not necessarily follow that since I own my gametes, I may therefore sell them. This is clearly not true with organs, though the same concept of ownership can be applied to them. The fact that a person does receive some compensation for sperm and egg donation, however, is consistent with the idea that he/she owns the sperm/eggs. When people anonymously donate sperm and eggs, they do so with the understanding that they are also relinquishing any parental claims on the child that will result from their donation. In other words, the genetic parents are the ones that initially hold parental rights, since they "own" the gametes. These rights can be surrendered upon donation of genetic materials.

In surrogacy, however, the contracting couple, whose egg and sperm are used, are not donating their gametes in the same way that anonymous donors do. They are clearly not relinquishing the parental rights that normally accompany one's genetic materials. They fully expect that they will be the legal and custodial parents of the child born out of the arrangement. Since they own their gametes, they thus have a claim on what becomes of their gametes when they are combined into a fertilized egg. This is similar to the way in which couples who undergo IVF own the embryos that are produced with their sperm and eggs. Prior to implantation in the surrogate, there is no dispute about to whom those embryos belong. In addition, they control the disposition of the embryos that are not implanted. If they "own" the embryos, then it follows that they also own the genetic materials necessary to produce them. It further follows that they have a priority claim on the child produced through the use of their genetic materials. This "ownership" may help explain the desire of infertile couples to have a child genetically related to them, and argues for the priority of genetics in determining motherhood.

In evaluating the claims of genetics in determining maternal

## JAPANESE GIRL BORN TO INDIAN SURROGATE ARRIVES HOME

A Japanese couple from Osaka utilized a fertility clinic in India for IVF treatment. An embryo created with the husband's sperm and an anonymous donor's egg was implanted into the womb of an Indian surrogate mother. However, the couple was divorced several months before the baby was born and the wife of the couple decided she no longer wanted the baby. Regardless, the Japanese father and grandmother traveled to India to pick up the child several months later. Under Indian law the mother of the baby must be present to receive a passport, but neither the Japanese mother nor the surrogate mother would cooperate. Since Indian law does not allow single men to adopt children, the father was unable to take his child home. After the story was spread through the media and the disputes continued, the baby was finally given a passport with just her Japanese father's name on it and was able to start her life with her family in Japan.

Source: "Japanese Girl Born to Indian Surrogate Arrives Home," March 29, 2010, CNN.com.

rights in surrogacy, there is little doubt about the influence of genetics in determining a person's identity and characteristics. A person's unique makeup comprises genetics, and sets him or her apart from any and all other individuals in the species. Genetic heritage surely is one of the strongest factors underlying the sense of bonding and connection felt between parent and child, and legitimately does motivate adopted children to go to substantial lengths to be reunited with their natural parents, often simply for the sake of being united.

### Intent to Parent as the Determinant of Motherhood

In an attempt to answer some of the difficult questions about parental rights in surrogacy and take into account the many possibilities offered by the new reproductive technologies, advocates of a new view of motherhood link parental rights with the preconception intent to become parents and raise the child produced by technologically assisted reproductive methods. This view of parental rights is known as "intent-based" parenthood.

The California Supreme Court majority opinion in the precedent-setting case for gestational surrogacy—*Johnson v. Calvert*—decided the case based partially on this view. The Court ruled that the preconception intent of the contracting couple should be the controlling factor in determining parental rights. They state, "Because two women each have presented acceptable claims of maternity, we do not believe that this case can be decided without enquiring into the parties' intentions as manifested in the surrogacy agreement. But for their [the Calverts'] acted-on intention, the child would not exist."[27] In effect, the Court used the preconception intent to become a parent as a "tiebreaker" when the biological contributions are divided among two women—the egg donor and the surrogate. Others want to see the intention to parent as the controlling factor in all surrogacy arrangements. We view that as very problematic, and see no reason why the intention to parent should necessarily be weighted more heavily than the biological factors.[28]

Preconception intent to parent has the appeal of simplicity in dealing with conflicts between the surrogate and the contracting couple, because it gives the intention, as expressed in the surrogacy contract, the status of a "trump card." But to give priority to intent in the determination of parental rights ignores critical biological realities. Intent needs biology for procreation to successfully occur, and frequently biology works in the absence of any intent to procreate. In addition, the notion of preconception intent to parent neglects the prospect that the surrogate may develop the intent to become a parent at some point in the process.

There is no reason why the surrogate's developing intent to parent should not be taken seriously since, when it does develop, she combines a biological contribution, a relationship with the child, and intent to parent, and thus possesses many of the critical components of motherhood. This aspect of developing intent to parent is widely recognized in adoption cases, and there is no reason why it should not also be recognized in surrogacy cases. We would suggest that the surrogate's developing intent to parent casts doubt on the use of the preconception intent as the tiebreaker in gestational surrogacy too, because there is no reason to weigh the preconception intent more heavily than the surrogate's developing intent to parent, since the latter is based on a very real bonding with the child she is carrying.

We would further argue that intent without biology contributes little to the creation of the objective entity known as a child. For example, and certainly not intending harshness, infertile couples who may have had the mental intent to conceive for years have made little tangible progress toward realizing their dreams of having a child, if they have not been able to make the biological connection between egg and sperm. Furthermore, biology can and does work in the absence of the intent to conceive. The myriad of unwanted pregnancies bears eloquent witness to biology working against the mental intent to conceive. Of course, in surrogacy, the intent to conceive is that which begins the entire process. But if artificial insemination or in vitro fertilization is not successful with the surrogate, the mental intent to conceive counts for very little in the actual realization of the couple's goal.

We both hold that a good argument can be made for either genetics or gestation as the determinant of motherhood, and are both skeptical about the importance of the preconception intent to parent. If you insisted that we take a position and asked us what the law should be on this—we would differ. I (Rae) lean more toward the position that gestation determines motherhood, that the woman who gives birth to the child is the mother. This is because of the "sweat equity" that she has in the child at the time of birth, in addition to the bonding, connection, and relationship that forms a real and tangible relationship that she has with the child she is carrying. By contrast, I (Riley) lean more toward the view that genetics determines motherhood, at least to the extent that the biological mother's name should appear on the birth certificate, even if it is listed separately from the legal parent's name. Both of us view surrogacy as a less than ideal alternative because it stands far outside God's original design for procreation occurring within the sacred context of marriage.

However, we also acknowledge that there are situations in which surrogacy would be acceptable, in those scenarios in which there is a conflict between the prima facie norm of procreation within marriage and the biblical commitment to the sanctity of life. For example, I (Rae) had a couple in my office some time ago who had had a very unfortunate experience with IVF. They had been trying to achieve pregnancy for roughly six years, and finally conceived triplets through IVF. Tragically, all three babies miscarried at roughly the fifth month of the pregnancy, and in the process the woman suffered a massive uterine hemorrhage, nearly died, and had to have an emergency hysterectomy. The couple was devastated with this outcome, but continued to be hopeful about having a child, since they still had five embryos left in storage from IVF.

Had she been able, she would have gladly implanted the remaining embryos herself (probably at two different times) and tried again to have a child. But her options were more limited due to her hysterectomy. She could discard the embryos, which she rightly saw was wrong and didn't want to do that anyway. She could donate the embryos to another couple, which they saw as pointless, since they still had a strong desire to be parents to their children they had conceived through IVF. Or they could hire a surrogate to carry the embryos for them.

In our view, the mandate to uphold the sanctity of life suggests that a rescue of these embryos is of utmost importance. One way to rescue these embryos would be to put them up for adoption. But normally couples don't do that unless their "quiver" of children is full (Ps. 127:5), and given the desirable continuity between procreation and parenting, this suggests that the option to raise their genetic children themselves ought to be weighted more heavily than the option to give them up for adoption. The only way to preserve the sanctity of life for the embryos and maintain the continuity between procreation and parenting would be to employ a surrogate to assist in the rescue of the couple's embryos. Though not ideal and far from the original design, due to the reality of life in a fallen world, we would hold that this was an acceptable use of surrogacy to facilitate a rescue and enable a couple to have a child. However, we do not want to see surrogacy as just another reproductive choice in the fertility arsenal.

## In Conclusion

Surrogacy presents some of the most vexing issues in the entire field of assisted reproductive technology. We have argued that surrogacy is at variance with the prima facie norm of God's design that procreation occur within the context of marriage. Surrogacy is at least, if not more, as intrusive to the marital bond as use of gamete donors. As a result, the law sometimes has to get involved to settle complicated matters of parental rights.

We suggested that some cases of surrogacy are more clear than others, that in cases of commercial, genetic surrogacy, baby-selling occurs, and it is possible that a woman could be denied the right to associate with her child. We also argued that in most forms of surrogacy, there is a concern about the potential for exploitation of the surrogate, and in all forms of surrogacy, there is the fear that comes from the surrogate needing to emotionally disassociate herself from the child she is carrying. We also took up the complex matter of the definition of motherhood in cases where the biological contribution is split between the egg donor and the surrogate. Here Dr. Riley and I have somewhat different views—she leans toward genetics as the determinant of motherhood, and I lean toward gestation. Both of us realize that this particular issue is not clear-cut and both of us are open to other arguments from the opposing view. We agree that there are some occasions when surrogacy is acceptable—when necessary as a part of a rescue of embryos that would otherwise be discarded.

*The ability to look into the womb and examine the genetic structure of tiny fetuses and even smaller embryos ultimately comes from God.*

# CHAPTER EIGHT

# Prenatal Genetic Testing

D r. Henderson, a geneticist, will see three couples this morn-ing, all referred because of concerns about bearing children.[1] Each couple is unique, as is each of the concerns, but there are common themes, too. The most apparent commonality is that fact that they each walk through the doors of Dr. Henderson's office: genetic testing is increasingly sought.

## Tim and Barbara

Tim and Barbara are about to have their first experience with genetic testing and counseling. They married in their midthirties and because of their ages, started trying to become pregnant shortly after their honeymoon. As is more common with couples their age, it took some time before they finally achieved a pregnancy. Barbara is now thirty-eight and three months pregnant with their first child. They are thrilled that she is expecting, but understandably concerned about what they have heard are the higher risks of their child being born with certain genetic abnormalities such as Down syndrome.

Barbara is aware that the possibility of having a child with Down syndrome increases with the age of the mother, and especially after age thirty-five. She is more than just aware—her younger sister, Suzie, has Down syndrome. Although Suzie is high functioning, Barbara knows several people with Down syndrome who are more severely affected.

Barbara is anxious to have the testing done, and is worried about the results. What if the tests show her child to have Down syndrome, or some other abnormality? She has some reservations about bringing a severely deformed child into the world, both for the sake of the child and for her and her husband's sake. She has told Tim that she would consider ending the pregnancy if the tests reveal genetic abnormalities in their child. If you were her friend and she came to you for your counsel, what would you tell her about the wisdom of this genetic testing and her plans based on the results of the tests?

### Dave and Diane

Dave and Diane will also be in Dr. Henderson's office today. Dave's family medical history includes some individuals who have suffered from Huntington's, a progressively degenerative neurological disease. It is a late onset genetic disease, with symptoms usually appearing when the person reaches thirty to forty years of age. Dave's father died in an auto accident at age thirty-five, and was not known to be affected, but he apparently had the gene, for Dave's test is positive.

Huntington's disease is an autosomal dominant trait—you only need one copy of the gene to develop the disease. If a parent has the disease, his or her child has a 50 percent chance of having the gene, too. Understandably, Dave and Diane are very concerned about the welfare of any children that they might have. Dave knows about the ravages of the disease: he has done his own research, but mostly, he saw it in his grandfather.

Both he and Diane are fairly sure that they do not want to subject a child to the horrors of Huntington's disease. But they want children very badly, and so far they are not comfortable with either adoption or a sperm donor that would enable them to bypass Dave's genes and still have children. In order to ensure the best probability of a child without the gene for Huntington's disease, they have decided to do a much more sophisticated form of prenatal genetic testing; it is called Preimplantation Genetic Diagnosis (PGD). They are going to test for the gene before Diane even becomes pregnant.

The way they can do this is by using in vitro fertilization instead of natural conception. Even though they do not have a known infertility problem, they think that it would make sense to have conception occur outside the womb. They will go through the procedure of having her eggs harvested and fertilized in the lab with his sperm. The resulting embryos will be tested to see which ones do not have the gene. Only the embryos that do not have the defective gene will be implanted; the ones that do have it will be discarded. This way they ensure that the child who develops in her womb will not have to grow up to be afflicted with Huntington's disease. It will help to have a number of embryos from which to choose, since some will likely have the gene and others may be damaged or destroyed in the process of testing them for the gene. If you were friends with this couple, how would you advise them about this kind of prenatal genetic testing?

### *Jim and Lori*

The third couple in the geneticist's office today is Jim and Lori. They have three boys, and they very much want a girl. In fact, the only reason they are trying to have a fourth child is that they might have a girl. They don't particularly want a larger family but they figure that all the additional expense and effort of a four-child family would be worth it to have a girl. They are opposed to abortion and to discarding embryos, so they are not open to aborting or to testing embryos.

However, they are interested in a new technology that would enable them to select gender prior to conception with a sperm sorting technology called MicroSort. They realize that this does not guarantee that they would have a girl but would greatly increase their chances of having a girl. If Jim and Lori were your friends, how would you advise them on this type of reproductive technology being used to select for gender?

### Choosing to Screen

The reasoning behind the push for genetic testing is exemplified by the following example. The American College of Obstetricians and Gynecologists' Committee on Genetics reaffirmed in 2007 that couples should be screened for cystic fibrosis prior to conception. Such screening allows couples to know their risk for having an affected child, they opined. This, in turn, allows the couples to consider a number of reproductive options, including genetic testing prior to implantation or prenatally, or even the use of donor gametes.[2] Unmentioned yet understood in the reproductive choices is the abortion of affected individuals. Bearing and rearing an affected child, or adoption, are neither choices that are mentioned nor recommended.

As couples consider the prospect of genetic testing, there are several questions to ask.

1. Why are we seeking genetic testing?
2. What kind of information do we want?
3. What will we do with the information once received?

## Different Types of Testing

Screening for genetic and other types of fetal defects has become increasingly a routine part of a pregnant woman's maternity care. The term *screening* implies testing to find evidence of a problem. Results of screening may lead to further tests to *diagnose* a condition. Sometimes, the line between screening and diagnosis is not clear. There are multiple tests available related to pregnancy and childbearing. These are generally described below.

## Ultrasound

Almost every pregnant woman with adequate prenatal care receives ultrasound images of her uterus and the fetus growing inside it. This is usually the first "picture" the couple has of their developing child. Ultrasounds are normally done around the sixteenth to eighteenth weeks of pregnancy. As the pregnancy progresses, the image of the fetus becomes clearer, until late in the pregnancy when the fetus is too large to be viewed well. The gender of the child is usually apparent to the trained eye, and some anomalies can be detected through ultrasound (and numerous abnormalities can be ruled out). One area of interest on the ultrasound is the area of the back of the fetus's neck, the nuchal area. This area is evaluated for abnormality, the so-called nuchal translucency screen.[3] An enlarged area of lucency, or clear space, here can be associated with Down syndrome, or it could be one

---

### GENDER SELECTION AND GENETIC TESTING

In 2008 the Human Fertilization and Embryology Act was written to prohibit sex selection for non-medical reasons. In contrast, in Professor Stephen Wilkinson's new book *Choosing Tomorrow's Children: The Ethics of Selective Reproduction*, he argues that gender selection should not be prohibited. In the same way that parents encourage children to grow into a person with certain characteristics, we can and should influence the future population by selecting which possible future children we produce in the first place. According to Wilkinson the only reasons to prohibit the use of reproductive technology for gender selection or screening for diseases and disability is if there is a serious imbalance of genders or if the decision is motivated by sexist attitudes or beliefs. Wilkinson's book addresses ethical questions regarding the use of medicine for health versus enhancement, and the ethical implications of modern-day uses of biotechnology.

Source: "Bioethics Expert: Parents Should Be Allowed to Use Selective Reproduction In Choosing Future Child's Gender," *The Medical News*, Feb. 27, 2010, News-Medical.Net.

of a few other abnormalities that cause thickening of the neck.

## Blood Tests

Maternal blood tests that can indicate a variety of fetal abnormalities constitute another routine method of testing. One in particular is the alphafetoprotein (AFP) test. A high level of AFP in the mother's blood can indicate that this key protein is leaking from the fetus into the mother's blood, suggesting that the fetus has a neural tube defect. These include such conditions as anencephaly, the failure of the fetus to develop any cerebral cortex in the brain; or spina bifida, an opening in the sac that surrounds the spinal cord. The severity of the damage to the spine and nervous system depends upon where the opening is along the spinal column and how large it is. Normally, the closer to the brain the opening, the more nerve damage will result. Since the test was initially developed, it has been refined to correct the high number of false positives and negatives. Considered routine for pregnant women, it is a much more reliable test today than it was initially. Some states, such as California, require doctors by law to offer the AFP test to all their maternity patients. Additionally, AFP, when combined with the results of other blood tests like inhibin A, human Chorionic Gonadotropin (hCG), and estriol, can aid in the diagnosis of Down syndrome.

Testing maternal blood for fetal abnormality can also be done through a test called a microarray, although this is not done routinely. The microarray can test more than 600,000 single nucleotide peptides (SNPs)—representing portions of the DNA—for genetic abnormalities. Even at this level, there are some limitations of this test, and certainly, the test results will require interpretation by highly trained counselors. Another application of blood tests is the use of genetic testing of would-be parents, such as Dave underwent. Some ramifications of genetic testing will be discussed later on in this chapter.

## Invasive Tests

A third type of prenatal test is usually reserved for women who are considered at higher risk for fetal abnormalities. Often, these are women who are older or who have a family history that would indicate a higher likelihood of defect being passed along to the child. This test is an amniocentesis and is normally done somewhere between the weeks sixteen to twenty-two of pregnancy. Amniocentesis is much more invasive for the mother and can be risky for both mother and fetus. Occasionally—a risk of 1/300, typically[4]—amniocentesis causes a miscarriage.

During development, the fetus normally sloughs off cells into the surrounding amniotic fluid in which the fetus is swimming. Some of these cells can be obtained through an amniocentesis. Guided by ultrasound to guard against injuring the fetus, the physician inserts a needle into the woman's abdomen and draws out some of the amniotic fluid. In the laboratory, the fetal cells from the amniotic fluid are analyzed to determine if the developing fetus has any genetic anomalies.

Another invasive prenatal test is called chorionic villus sampling (CVS). This test, too, captures some of the fetus's cells but gets them from a different place. The chorionic villi make up the edges of the placenta, and they look like a cluster of small hairs that surround the sides of the placenta. The physician will obtain the chorionic villi through the cervix with a catheter, or, if necessary due to the location of the placenta, either through the woman's abdomen, similar to amniocentesis. Because this procedure, when done at nine to ten weeks of pregnancy, was associated with limb reduction (abnormalties in the hands, feet, arms, or legs[5]), this test is now typically performed about the twelfth to thirteenth weeks of pregnancy. The risk of fetal loss is approximately 1/200 for this procedure.[6] Should a couple find out that their child has abnormalities and they do not want to continue the pregnancy, it is emotionally easier on some couples to terminate the pregnancy in the first rather than the second trimester.

## PGS: Preimplantation Genetic Screening

There is now testing that can be done on embryos prior to the time a pregnancy is achieved. Embryos obtained through IVF can be evaluated for abnormalities prior to implantation so only the embryos that are without known genetic defects are candidates for implantation. It is usually done at the eight-cell stage of embryo development; one of the cells, called a blastomere, is taken from the embryo for testing. Since all the cells at that point are capable of developing into all cell types of the body, the subtraction of one cell does not appear to usually cause problems for the embryo, although there is a risk associated with the procedure. That risk was estimated in 2004:

> Lawrence Werlin, leading fertility researcher and cofounder of the GENESYS (Gender in Economic and Social Systems Project) Network for Reproductive Health, argues that risks associated with the embryo biopsy process of PGD can be reduced significantly through good laboratory technique. "In controlled situations, where people are used to doing embryo biopsies and blastomere fixation, your risk of having a false negative would be very low, and your chance of damaging the embryo is probably in the region of 5%, while the risk of embryos arresting due to the PGD is probably 5% to 10%."[7]

Preimplantation Genetic Screening (PGS) involves taking a cell from the developing embryo and checking it for an abnormal chromosome number. Normal chromosome number for humans is forty-six, including a set of sex chromosomes. Females have two X chromosomes, while males have one X and one Y sex chromosome. PGS is often offered to women who have had repeated pregnancy losses or IVF failures, or women of advanced age. According to the Genetics and Public Policy Center, "More than two-thirds of in vitro fertilization (IVF) clinics offer preimplantation genetic screening (PGS), even though most clinic directors believe that more research is needed to determine when—or even whether—the technique should be offered to patients."[8]

In PGD, embryos are tested for specific genetic conditions or traits, and only those that do not have the undesirable condition, or do have

## PREIMPLANTATION GENETIC DIAGNOSIS OVERSOLD, SAY IVF EXPERTS

The number of people receiving preimplantation genetic diagnosis (PGD), also called genetic screening, at IVF clinics grew significantly in Europe from 1998 to 2007. PGD is used in IVF clinics to screen for genetic diseases and choose the sex of the babies. However, researchers believe the increased use of the service is due to an incorrect claim that PGD is a surer way to conceive a child for older mothers or for women having trouble with miscarriages. In response, the European Society of Human Reproduction and Embryology stated that there is no reason to believe PGD is helpful for older women or women who have had repeated miscarriages. Such procedures should only be used when there is scientific reason to do so, not because it is popular or falsely advertised.

Source: Michael Cook. "Preimplantation Genetic Diagnosis Oversold, Say IVF Experts," *BioEdge*, March 20, 2010, bioedge.org.

the desirable traits, are implanted. Thus, embryos with certain muscular dystrophies may not be implanted; conversely, those embryos that perfectly match a sibling's blood and tissue type may be chosen. These are both possibilities with PGD.

## The Human Genome Project

One of the primary reasons for prenatal genetic testing becoming more widespread is that the amount of genetic information available to couples has increased exponentially in the past few years. This is primarily the result of a project called the Human Genome Project, an enormous worldwide effort designed to map the entire human genetic code.[9]

The project, the first draft of which was published in 2001, has as its goal identifying which genes are responsible for which traits in the human genetic code. Researchers are discovering heretofore unknown (but suspected in many cases) genetic links with numerous diseases, or at least predispositions to certain diseases. For example, genetic links to numerous cancers, heart disease, mental illness, and other debilitating diseases were discovered in the course of the project. Once a specific link or predisposition is pinpointed to a specific gene, then a diagnostic test can often be developed to enable a couple to have prenatal testing done (the testing can also be done for adults). The project promises to produce an abundance of genetic information

## GENETIC NONDISCRIMINATION ACT OF 2008

The statute defines "genetic information" as information about:

an individual's genetic tests (including genetic tests done as part of a research study); genetic tests of the individual's family members (defined as dependents and up to and including 4th degree relatives); genetic tests of any fetus of an individual or family member who is a pregnant woman, and genetic tests of any embryo legally held by an individual or family member utilizing assisted reproductive technology; the manifestation of a disease or disorder in family members (family history); any request for, or receipt of, genetic services or participation in clinical research that includes genetic services (genetic testing, counseling, or education) by an individual or family member. Genetic information does not include information about the sex or age of any individual.

The statute defines "genetic test" as an analysis of human DNA, RNA, chromosomes, proteins, or metabolites that detects genotypes, mutations, or chromosomal changes. The results of routine tests that do not measure DNA, RNA, or chromosomal changes, such as complete blood counts, cholesterol tests, and liver-function tests, are not protected under GINA. Also, under GINA, genetic tests do not include analyses of proteins or metabolites that are directly related to a manifested disease, disorder, or pathological condition that could reasonably be detected by a health care professional with appropriate training and expertise in the field of medicine involved.

Source: Department of Health and Human Services (HHS), "'GINA,' The Genetic Information Nondiscrimination Act of 2008: Information for Researchers and Health Care Professionals," April 6, 2009, genome.gov/Pages/PolicyEthics/GeneticDiscrimination/GINAInfoDoc.pdf.

that can be used by couples who wish to know what genetic predispositions their child has inherited. Of course, certain conditions have well-known genetic links, such as Down syndrome and Huntington's disease, but the number of conditions for which a fetus can be tested has dramatically increased as a result of the genome project. In 2003, there were nine hundred genetic tests possible;[10] in 2010, more than two thousand genetic tests were available.[11]

Though the project raises the long-term prospect of engineering for genetic enhancement, the more immediate promise of the project is the information it will provide. Some conditions can be treated in utero through the exciting field of fetal therapy. But in many cases, the information available to the couple will help them prepare for their child. In some cases, what a couple finds out about their child will likely result in their terminating the pregnancy.

Couples undergoing prenatal testing are not the only ones interested in this information. Employers and insurance carriers may also be interested. For that reason, the Genetic Information Nondiscrimination Act of 2008 (GINA) was passed. It does not apply to everyone in every circumstance, but generally prohibits genetic discrimination in health insurance and employment. Exactly how it will be applied, regulated, and enforced is not yet clear, but the principle of genetic nondiscrimination is clear.

Back to the worried expecting couple, for whom a whole new world of information is opening up. The Genome Project may make genetic testing more routine because the number of conditions that are detectable in the womb is rapidly increasing. In the past, genetic testing was primarily for those couples whose family history indicated some possibility of a genetic disease. But in the future, with numerous fairly inexpensive diagnostic tests available for a wide range of genetic conditions, such testing may become more routine.

There seems to be little doubt about the potential demand for testing. Of all the questions that prospective parents ask when they find out they are pregnant, such as "Is it a boy or girl?," "Who will the baby look like?" "What will his temperament be?" "Will she be an easy baby?" the most anxiety-producing question is no doubt: "Will the baby be healthy?" This desire for reassurance about the baby's health gnaws at most parents-to-be and drives them to genetic testing and genetic counselors if they have concerns.

## The Ethics of Prenatal Genetic Testing

### Gaining Information

In the biblical and theological framework for reproductive technologies that was laid out in part I, one of the conclusions drawn was that medical technology generally improves the lot of the human race and helps alleviate effects of the entrance of sin into the world—and that its doing so is an aspect of God's general revelation.

The ability of human beings to look into the womb and examine the genetic structure of tiny fetuses, and even smaller embryos, ultimately comes from God. His wisdom revealed outside of Scripture has enabled human beings to develop the technology that identifies the results of the Fall in the form of genetic diseases.[12]

Thus prenatal genetic testing per se does not appear to be wrong. That does not suggest necessarily that couples are morally obligated to use the available testing technology. It is important that couples acknowledge that the womb is still "the secret place" over which God alone ultimately has control (Ps. 139:15).

Further, they should realize that these tests are not infallible (all have some margin of error, greater for some than others) and some do involve a degree of risk both to the mother and the fetus. In addition, the degree of abnormality can be difficult to predict based solely on the genetic test. If the benefit of obtaining the information is greater than or proportionate to the risk incurred in the test, then utilizing genetic testing technology is morally appropriate.

### Using Information

What couples do with the information gleaned from prenatal genetic testing is, however, quite another matter. Most genetic counselors will say that they operate with the presumption of objectivity. Their role is to give information and maximize reproductive choice for the couple.[13] Yet when public health officials talk about the benefits of prenatal screening in reducing the incidence of genetic diseases, that discussion often assumes that couples will end their pregnancy if they receive bad news from their testing.[14]

In some of the medical literature in this area, the term "amniocentesis" is used to refer to the process not only of the testing but also of the abortion that the authors assume a couple will authorize if their fetus is discovered to have some genetic defect.[15] The suggestion is often made that prenatal testing is a great help in eliminating the incidence of genetic diseases. But the only way prenatal testing can eliminate genetic or chromosomal disorders is if couples end their pregnancies. Genetic disease is thus being eliminated, but preemptively, and at the expense of the child who has the disease. It is one thing to decrease the incidence of these genetic diseases, but quite another to do so by eliminating the person who has the disease.

The incidence of every disease would decrease dramatically if medicine had the liberty to do away with the people who have it. There is a difference between finding a solution to a problem and eliminating the problem. In many genetic counseling offices, there is an assumption that if testing comes back indicating genetic defects, the couple will end the pregnancy. Couples who utilize prenatal genetic testing should be aware of this assumption prior to the start of the testing.

This abortion assumption is certainly understandable. Couples who discover that their child has a genetic abnormality are often understandably pulled by the desire to end their pregnancy. After the anticipation of conception and the excitement of pregnancy, to find out that the child you are carrying has genetic defects can be a crushing disappointment that many couples wish to put behind them by ending the pregnancy. In addition, couples want to avoid the difficult scenario of rearing a handicapped child with all of the attendant physical, emotional, and financial demands.

However, the difficulty of going through with an abortion of a genetically deformed fetus should not be underestimated either. Most genetic anomalies are detected by amniocentesis or other tests that are performed, and the results obtained, in the second trimester of pregnancy. By this time the fetus is beginning to resemble a baby and its features are becoming more pronounced and visible by ultrasound. This is not to say that the appearance of humanness is a valid criterion for the right to life, but rather, that the more the fetus resembles a baby, the more emotionally difficult it is in many cases for the parents to authorize the abortion. Many couples experience profound grief, loss, and guilt when abortion for deformity is performed.

## Tough Calls

Ultimately what counts the most is not the emotional element involved in the decision to terminate a pregnancy when the fetus is genetically defective. What matters is what reason and Scripture have to say about the personhood of the unborn. If it is true that the fetus is a person and the result of a continuous process of development that begins at conception, in which there is no metaphysically relevant decisive moment, then the fetus, irrespective of the stage of development it is in, is deserving of all the rights to life. The problematic element in prenatal genetic testing is the decision to end a pregnancy because of the information that the testing reveals.

The presence of a genetically deformed child in the womb is often used to justify abortion. There is no doubt that finding out that one's child in utero is not healthy is a difficult situation with which to deal. It is important to analyze the decision to end a pregnancy because of genetic anomalies and how it is justified.

The most frequent justification is by a quality of life argument. This argument states that the child born with such abnormalities is deemed incapable of having a life worth living. The child will never grow up to be what a normal child would be in terms of mental capacity, and in some cases will not even have normal bodily functions. In many cases the child will have a life filled with suffering. For example, children with severe Down syndrome or spina bifida (a hole in the sac that protects the spinal cord, causing nervous system damage) end up with very difficult lives, for the most part incapable of meaningful interaction and function.

In some more extreme and very severe cases such as anencephaly (a condition in which the child is born with the majority of its brain missing: only the brain stem, which controls the involuntary functions, is present), the argument is sometimes made that the child is so deformed that it cannot properly be called a person, and thus has no rights to life.

### Guidelines for Making Decisions

Testing results that indicate a genetic anomaly in a couple's child, however, do not justify ending the pregnancy, for a number of reasons. First, the couple must realize that these tests do have a margin of error. They are not infallible and should not be taken by the couple as error-free. Errors can be either false positives or false negatives. Abnormal test results may require involved follow-up testing and produce substantial anxiety to the couple who is awaiting the results. Even amniocentesis is not 100 percent reliable. Couples should be very careful about terminating a pregnancy based on tests that can be in error.

Second, assuming that the tests are entirely accurate, the degree of deformity that the child will experience is difficult to predict. For example, there are varying degrees of abnormality with Down syndrome. Some cases are very severe while others are quite mild. Those with mild cases often lead relatively normal lives and are virtually indistinguishable to the casual observer. Symptoms of some genetic diseases such as Huntington's disease have an onset later in life. Until the symptoms develop, the person lives an entirely normal life, usually until sometime between the ages of thirty and forty.

Third, assuming that the degree of deformity experienced can be predicted with certainty, it is presumptuous to suggest that the lives of the genetically or otherwise disabled are not worth living. That is a value judgment, not a medical fact, and no one, including parents, however well-meaning, should have the right to impose that kind of value judgment upon another person, especially when doing so results in their death.

In many cases like these in which abortion is contemplated, the parents likely confuse the burden of life for the child with the burden of caring for the child as the parents. The life that is not worth living is not that of the child but of the parent, having to care for such a child. Though society should not underestimate the challenge of a lifetime of caring for these children, the notion of a life not worth living for the child should not be used to disguise what is often the real reason the child is being aborted, because of the burden on the parents. The hardship on the parents does not justify ending the pregnancy, any more than the financial hardship of a poor woman justifies her ending her pregnancy. Although this stance may sound harsh, it is actually a recognition of the fact that our lives are to be lived in community. Such realities place a call upon the church and community to provide support and care, to "bear one another's burdens."

It is further presumptuous to suggest that the life of the genetically handicapped fetus is not worth living. There is no inherent connection between disability and unhappiness; nor is there any intrinsic link between disability and personal fulfillment. It would interesting to take an informal and anecdotal survey of handicapped individuals and ask them if, on account of their disability, they viewed their life as not worth living and would have preferred never to have been born at all. We would surely find that unhappiness does not necessarily follow from having a handicap. Some of the most fulfilled and happy people we have met are those who have succeeded in overcoming their disabilities, and they would likely be offended at the suggestion that their lives are "unhappy," not to mention "not worth living."

A fourth and the most important reason that handicap does not justify ending a pregnancy is that the entity in the womb, however genetically deformed, is still a human person. Those who defend the moral right of parents to abort genetically defective children assume, whether acknowledged or not, that the fetus is less than a full human person. One has to hold such an assumption in order for this justification of abortion to make any sense. For if the handicapped unborn is a person, then this justification of abortion is absurd. Unless one assumes that the handicapped unborn is not a person, there is no morally significant difference between abortion for reasons of genetic deformity and executing adults who are genetically handicapped. Yet very few consider executing handicapped adults simply on the basis of their handicap, for the simple reason that society acknowledges that they are persons with the right to life. In fact, the handicapped are deemed more worthy of protection from discrimination, not less, because of their vulnerability due to the physical and/or mental challenges they face. If the fetus, irrespective of genetic defect is a person, then the decision to abort based on such defect cannot be justified. Surely it is better to suffer the tragedy of accepting a child with genetic abnormalities than to inflict suffering on another person by abortion.[16]

## When It's Terminal

Some particularly severe anomalies may seem inconsistent with the child being a person. For example, a child with anencephaly, perhaps the most severe abnormality with which a child can be born, will have no ability to do anything except maintain essential bodily functions. The child is born with only a brain stem, and has no cerebral part of the brain. Thus the child will have no sense of self-consciousness, no awareness of his or her environment, and no ability to interact or form any kind of human relationships. For many people, the decision to abort an anencephalic child is an easy one, and many medical professionals have concluded that anencephalics are not persons because they are so deformed.[17] But simply because the child does not have the capacity to perform certain functions, it does not follow that the child is not a person. Functional definitions of personhood are both metaphysically inconsistent and socially potentially dangerous.[18] Personhood is a matter of essence, not function.

Admitting that the anencephalic child is a person, however, does not by itself mean that all treatment to save his/her life once born is appropriate. An anencephalic child is essentially born with a terminal illness. Most anencephalics die within the first month of life, though some do live for as long as a year. There is no obligation to treat a terminally ill patient when the treatment is futile, that is, it would not improve the patient's condition and help restore the person to health. Since the anencephalic child is for the most part imminently dying from birth, there is no obligation to offer aggressive medical treatment. Of course, for all dying patients, there is the obligation to provide comfort and dignity care, that is, care that maintains their comfort and dignity while allowing the disease to take its natural course. Thus, one does not have to deny personhood to the anencephalic child in order to justify not providing aggressive treatment.

Then one can ask, "If it is legitimate to provide only comfort and dignity care for anencephalics and let their condition take its natural course, then why is it not acceptable to end the pregnancy?" Continuing a pregnancy of an anencephalic baby is a troublesome and emotionally arduous situation. But we are hesitant to endorse ending such a pregnancy for two reasons. First, there are at times questions about the diagnosis and the severity of the deformity that cannot be confirmed until after birth. Thus, it seems best to wait until after birth to make decisions about the care of the child instead of ending the pregnancy. Second, there is a significant moral difference between actively taking someone's life and passively allowing a natural death to occur. In the latter the cause of death is the disease or condition afflicting the child, but in the former, the cause of death is actually the action of the physician performing the abortion.[19]

## To Test or Not to Test?

If couples do not accept the abortion assumption underlying much prenatal genetic testing, then it would seem to be an appropriate technology that they can utilize. But if a couple is committed to continuing the pregnancy regardless of the results of the tests, then one might ask, "What is the purpose for having the testing done in the first place?" It would seem pointless and perhaps even foolish to submit to the risks of some of these tests when the results will not affect the decision about continuing the pregnancy. Certainly in some cases that is true and it would be unwise to undergo the riskier tests without a compelling reason to do so. However, it is legitimate to use prenatal genetic testing to prepare for the arrival of a child who will end up having a genetic defect.

There does not seem to be any good reason not to have the tests that carry little risk and are not invasive, such as ultrasound imaging and certain blood tests, such as the tri- or quad-screen offered by most obstetricians. In fact, for most couples, seeing their child on the ultrasound monitor for the first time is a treasured experience. The ultrasound image can usually identify the gender of the child if the parents desire to know that prior to birth. If there are good reasons such as a family history of genetic disease or advanced age of the mother to indicate further genetic testing, then these too are legitimate if used either to reassure the parents that their child is healthy, or to prepare them—emotionally and perhaps financially—for the rigors of rearing a handicapped child. Even couples who have a strong preference for one gender over another, for whatever the reason, would be well served by ultrasound and disclosure of the child's gender. This may be the case with a couple who has a number of children of the same gender and desire the next child to be a different sex (so-called family balancing). If the child is not of the desired gender, then the parents have time to work through the disappointment prior to the delivery date. By the time of the child's birth, they are emotionally prepared to bond properly with that newborn child—bonding that is crucial to the child's development.

In addition, there are some genetic anomalies that can be treated if care is initiated shortly after birth or even in the womb. For example, with spina bifida, physicians have traditionally closed the sac surrounding the spinal column after birth. To do this, the child must go immediately from the delivery room to the operating room, minimizing the exposure to the spinal column. It is very helpful to everyone concerned if this condition is known prior to birth. However, the field of fetal therapy is developing some exciting technologies that enable physicians to treat some conditions and even perform surgery on developing fetuses in the womb. This is the case with spina bifida today, as the condition can be corrected in utero. As the field of fetal surgery continues to grow, more conditions will likely be treatable in utero, contributing to further legitimate demand for prenatal testing.

## To Sum Up

Use of prenatal genetic testing is morally legitimate when used to

### BABY SAMUEL'S SPINA BIFIDA SURGERY

At 21 weeks gestation, baby Samuel Armas had surgery, from inside his mother's womb. Samuel had prenatal surgery to correct spina bifida, thereby closing the sac that protects the spinal cord. Surgeon Dr. Joseph Bruner performed the delicate surgery, and had the remarkable reaction of the baby actually reaching out and grabbing his finger with his tiny hand. Photographer Michael Clancy recorded the event on film and has some touching photos of the baby's hand protruding out of the womb. Some surgeons maintain that this kind of invasive surgery may be unnecessary some day, when stem cell treatments in utero may be preferred.

Source: Cassandra Willard, "Tinkering in the Womb," *Nature Medicine* 14 (2008): 1176-77, available at http://www.nature.com/nm/journal/v14/n11/full/nm1108-1176.html. For the photos, the source is www.michaelclancy.com.

obtain information about the child in utero in order to prepare the parents for care of this child and, if necessary, prepare physicians for appropriate treatment of the child. That is the proper use of the information gleaned from the testing. To use the results to authorize and justify ending the pregnancy is not legitimate since the parents would be condemning the handicapped unborn to death simply on the basis of its genetic anomaly. The only way this can be justified is to assume that the fetus with inherited abnormalities is less than a fully human person, an assumption that cannot be maintained. But if the handicapped unborn is indeed a person, then ending a pregnancy on the basis of the handicap is the most vicious form of discrimination.

## PGD—Genetic Testing of Preimplantation Embryos

Technological progress now provides the possibility of testing embryos prior to implantation—before pregnancy. The DNA structure of the embryo can now be analyzed to check for any genetic abnormalities. This technology has developed quickly and quietly and is known as PGD (preimplantation genetic diagnosis).

### *What Is PGD For?*

PGD can only be done on IVF embryos. Thus, couples desirous of utilizing PGD must also use IVF, even if they are not infertile. They may be couples much like the two featured at the beginning of this chapter, who are interested in a particular genetic makeup of their potential child(ren). The defective embryos could be discarded instead of implanted and the couple would have greater assurance that their fetus would not carry any deleterious genes.

Some researchers see PGD as a means to move toward eliminating certain types of genetic diseases. One such statement, made by a fertility clinic medical director, was reported in a 2004 article: "PGD may well introduce new, as yet unknown risks at the same time as eliminating known genetic or chromosomal disorders, but more work needs to be done."[20] Others see it as a first step in actually correcting such defects through genetic engineering. In the same way that physicians can treat some defects in utero through fetal therapy, it may be possible in the future to treat some conditions through embryo therapy.

## *Evaluating the Use of PGDs*

Though PGD sounds like a responsible way for couples with a history of genetic abnormalities to procreate, there is more to it than that. If personhood begins at conception, then there is no moral difference between aborting a fetus and discarding an embryo. If the results of genetic testing indicate that certain embryos are defective, then there is no moral difference between discarding them and aborting defective fetuses (and for that matter, executing handicapped adults).[21] In addition, in the process of testing the embryos, they are sometimes unintentionally damaged and then are discarded, and this is problematic for the same reason that research that damages the embryo is a problem. In general, research on a human being that is not for the subject's benefit, is done without the subject's consent, and could likely lead to destruction of the research subject should not be allowed in society. Similarly, embryo testing that damages embryos or leads to their being discarded is morally problematic.

However, embryo testing for couples at risk for transmitting genetic diseases seems to be a very responsible way of procreating children. Rather than taking their chances with the roll of the genetic dice, using embryo testing gives them a measure of control and assures them of not passing on harmful genes to their child or children. To deny the legitimacy of embryo testing may seem to take away the only responsible way of procreating a genetically related child for couples who have a history of genetic disease.

However, the underlying reasoning that justifies embryo testing in this case is a crude form of utilitarianism, in which the ends justify the means, and in which moral principles are subservient to results. It is problematic for the results of any technology to be the moral

## PGD AND DESIGNER CHILDREN

Preimplantation Genetic Diagnosis (PGD) is used mostly as a screening for genetic diseases but is also available for a couple who wants to screen for eye color, hair color, and other physical traits. Instead of screening for genetic disease, or for gender, the couple screens for the trait or traits they desire. Embryos conceived through IVF are a necessary part of the process. Following the screening, the embryos with the desired traits are implanted and the remaining ones are either kept in storage, discarded, or donated to other infertile couples. Many bioethicists are concerned about the use of PGD for this purpose, calling it a distortion of the purpose of medicine. Others say that the decision about how to use this technology should be left up to parents and patients. Some prospective parents actually use PGD for selecting certain disabilities, such as deafness, thus intentionally creating a child with that disability. A Johns Hopkins University survey found that 3% of PGD clinics offered this "negative enhancement" service, while 42% of clinics offered gender selection services.

Sources: Gaugum Naik, "A Baby, Please. Blond, Freckles—Hold the Colic," *Wall Street Journal*, Feb. 12, 2009, online.wsj.com.
Ronald Bailey, "Hooray for Designer Babies," *Reason*, March 6, 2002, reason.com.

trump card that is the overriding consideration in determining the proper use of such a technology. Though one cannot help but have deep empathy for couples with a history of genetic disease, sacrificing embryonic persons for the sake of their having a healthy child is too high a cost for the Christian couple who holds that personhood begins at conception.

Of course, for the couple who denies the personhood of the unborn or holds that its personhood begins at some later point in pregnancy, this presents no moral dilemma and can be considered a responsible way to avert some of the risks of procreation.

## MicroSort and Gender Selection

Families sometimes prefer one gender over another, for a variety of reasons. In some parts of the world, males are preferred for many reasons, some of which involve discrimination against females. Or some families may be in the situation that Jim and Lori faced in the introduction to this chapter—they want to balance their family and have both genders among their children. They do not devalue either gender but have a preference for a balanced family.

As mentioned earlier, in the United States, a procedure known as MicroSort is available for sex selection, and its use is growing. The benefit of this technology is that it can be used prior to conception, and thus it makes both abortion and discarding embryos unnecessary. It can be used to exclude X-chromosome related disorders by excluding the X chromosome from the sperm, or for family balancing. Although not 100 percent successful, their results are striking.[22] Estimates are that use of MicroSort technology gives a better than 80 percent chance of conceiving the desired gender.

Testing for sex/gender selection for "social reasons" is normally opposed by most bioethics scholars,[23] but in clinics across the country, it occurs more frequently than one might suppose. Although it is rarely admitted that a couple is ending a pregnancy for that reason, it does happen in the United States and other parts of the West.

It occurs with alarming regularity in other countries where women's rights are not what they are in the West or where girls are not as highly valued as boys. For example, in India, where male children are valued much more than female, physicians and genetic counselors are in a difficult bind, wanting to offer the testing but fully aware that some couples will routinely end the pregnancy if testing reveals that the child is a girl. Similarly in China, males are preferred. China's family planning policy "stipulates that couples living in cities can have one child, unless one or both are from an ethnic minority or they are both only children. In most rural areas a couple may have a second child after a break of several years."[24] Sex-specific abortion of female fetuses is widespread;[25] infanticide of female newborns is sometimes practiced.[26]

The cultural results are problematic, as a study by the Chinese Academy of Social Sciences shows. "Authorities put the normal male-female ratio at between 103–107 males for every 100 females. But in 2005, the last year for which data were made available, there were 119 boys for every 100 girls. . . ."[27] Because of the abnormal ratio of males to females, it is estimated that by 2020, more than 24 million Chinese men will be without wives.[28] This is a major concern and suggests a significant problem when gender selection is viewed from the broader, societal perspective, particularly when there are social conditions that suggest it would be practiced on a widespread scale.

It seems clear that gender selection based on a bias against one gender is morally very problematic, both because of the discrimination and the social consequences it produces. But what about preconception gender selection in order to balance out one's family, when there is no obvious gender bias and no abortion or discarding of embryos? What would we say to Jim and Lori, whom you met in the introduction to this chapter, as they were wrestling with the desire to balance their family and the decision to use MicroSort?

One immediate question to put to couples like Jim and Lori is why they want to have a specific gender, and to discern if there are certain gender-specific expectations that accompany the desire to have a boy or girl. These kinds of noncharacter expectations can be potentially damaging to a child, and if the desire for a certain gender is driven by these expectations, we would discourage the couple from using MicroSort technology for this purpose.

More broadly, the Bible clearly indicates that children are a gift from God (Ps. 127:1–3) to be treasured and unconditionally loved. To be sure, in biblical times, children were a gift in that they were also economic assets, able to work in an agrarian society and care for aging parents when they became unable to work. But the notion of children as a gift suggests that they are to be received gratefully from the hand of God, *without specifications or conditions*. In

## MISSING GIRLS

In the Asia-Pacific region of the world the term "missing girls" refers to the estimated 100 million "missing" women who have died due to poor health care, neglect, infanticide, or abortion, ultimately all a product of sex selection. In a culture where girls are seen as less valuable than men, people use any means to abandon baby girls, and the ratio of men to women is growing larger each day. With so many men and a decline of women, the number of unmarried young men is on the rise. Further, there is a strong correlation between the number of unmarried young men and the rise in violence, making unmarried men a threat to society. Researchers claim that gender inequality is stifling potential social progress and justice of the region. The United Nations Development Program (UNDP) is working to change both the policies and the attitudes toward women in hopes that women will be treated and viewed equally, and there will be an end to the "missing girls."

Source: Marcy Darnovsky, "What Happens When Modern Reproductive Technology Meets Son Preference?" The Center for Genetics and Society, March 11, 2010, Psychologytoday. com/blog.

fact, wedding registries and Christmas lists excepted, we generally consider it inappropriate to put specifications on gifts we receive. And we surely question a person who takes matters into his or her own hands to ensure that the gift they are receiving is just exactly what they want. Though use of MicroSort cannot undermine God's sovereignty over the assignment of a child's gender, dependence on this technology can undercut a couple's trust in God's providence over them. We admit that neither of these points may be sufficient to argue definitively against preconception gender selection, but they should give substantial pause to the couple who is considering MicroSort technology.

## Social Concerns about Prenatal Testing

Beyond the clinical issues about when specifically prenatal genetic

testing is legitimate to use, there are other concerns about prenatal genetic testing in general. What kind of cultural ethos is being created
by the growing prevalence of this kind of testing and routine abortion
when the results are not what the couple desires? How is the growing
availability of prenatal testing affecting the way society thinks about
reproduction? Two potential effects of this growth in genetic testing
are worth further thought.

The first relates to how society views the disabled adult population. Disability advocacy groups are understandably concerned about
the abortion assumption inherent in a good deal of genetic testing.
They fear that the loss of respect for the disabled unborn will trans-
late into less respect for the adult disabled population. There is a curious double standard at work here. Virtually everyone writing on
medical ethics condemns abortion for the purpose of sex selection,
on the grounds that it makes a powerful statement about the relative
value of the female gender. Since most who contemplate sex selection favor boys, a preference that is overwhelmingly the case in much
of the third world and places where there are restrictive population
policies, feminist groups are rightly concerned about what that says
about the value of their gender in society. But when it comes to the
disabled, no such concern is apparent, since society has already sanctioned abortion for virtually any disability that the testing uncovers.[29]
We are content to draw our moral lines at gender but not at disability.

The President's Commission on Bioethics in the 1980s illustrates
this double standard. The commission gives approval for genetic testing; it also condemns use of such testing for sex selection. They state
that sex selection "is incompatible with the attitude of virtually unconditional acceptance that developmental psychologists have found to be
essential to successful parenting. For the good of all children, society's
efforts should go into promoting the acceptance of each individual—
with his or her particular strengths and weaknesses—rather than rein-
forcing the negative attitudes that lead to rejection."[30] What holds for
gender should also hold for disability. One can argue that the disabled,

because of their greater degree of vulnerability, are owed this acceptance even more so than healthy children, irrespective of gender.

This unconditional love and acceptance that are at the heart of all responsible parenthood may also be affected by the cultural ethos produced by widespread genetic screening. Testing can involve a conflict between unconditional love for a child and a parental desire to have the best for their children. Sociologist Barbara Katz Rothman asks pointedly, "What does it do to motherhood, to women, and to men as fathers too, when we make parental acceptance conditional, pending further testing. We ask the mother and her family to say in essence, 'These are my standards. If you meet these standards of acceptability, then you are mine and I will love you and accept you totally. After you pass this (genetic) test.'"[31]

The extreme form of this occurs in the futuristic scenarios in which parents use testing and genetic engineering to customize their children, by selecting the most desirable traits and gender. Though trait selection for children is still in the future, the mentality that underlies it may already be present. Though it is legitimate for parents to want every advantage for their children, seeking such advantage must not come at the expense of the unconditional acceptance that is what ultimately gives children their greatest advantage. To the degree that prenatal testing encourages a way of thinking that undercuts parental love and acceptance toward children, society should be very careful about endorsing its widespread use. This is one further reason why for the Christian, the morally acceptable use of testing should be for preparation, not abortion. Children and the disabled are already marginalized enough in Western culture. Society in general and individual couples in particular should be cautious about endorsing prenatal genetic testing if indeed it undermines one of the essentials of responsible parenthood.

# Afterword

As persons created in the image of our Creator God, we have more than a mere drive to reproduce—we possess an inherent desire to procreate. Our desire for children, therefore, is only natural considering our creative heritage. Moreover, the process by which we participate in God's creativity is awe-filled and nothing short of miraculous. The fruit of that partnership is a gift indeed.

But for many, this desire is often not readily fulfilled. While others seem to "pop out" babies without a second thought, for some couples years of effort have yielded empty arms, triggering prayerful pleas of "Why us?"

The journey of infertility is not for the fainthearted; it is long, arduous, and painful. Those who are Christians must strive to walk it faithfully and with spiritual integrity. We must take care that our desire to procreate does not deteriorate into mere reproduction. For in the end, the process of procreation is one over which we have little control. Herein lie the promise and hope—and danger—of reproductive technologies.

Technology is a gift of God's grace, but must be employed as such, in recognition that it is one to be utilized humbly, responsibly, and gratefully. As a gift, it offers hope and fulfillment to many couples. But as with any good thing, its misuse can have adverse ramifications: the panacea of reproductive technologies can inadvertently become a Pandora's box of long-term detrimental consequences. As good stewards of God's gracious gift, we must partner with God in its use, for technology is fraught with moral difficulties—difficulties that require reverent reflection and prayerful discernment. Such stewardship entails that we set limits before engaging these technologies and exhibit a willingness to accept children as a gift from God's hand rather than a product of our own. It involves exercising trust in a God who grants more than we can think or ask.

Our understanding of embryos as persons who are beginning a journey of their own, created and ordained by God, must be the primary principle governing our approach to the use of any technology. We must be careful not to wantonly destroy the lives we have helped to create.

Techniques aimed at restoration of function, in general, are morally permissible; but all techniques, even when permissible, can interfere with or even endanger the intimacy of the couple. This is a crucial risk, and one that must be carefully considered, for whether it involves a physician, donor, surrogate, or lawyer, at least one additional party is introduced into a relationship intended only for two. A loving process becomes mechanical and technical—often painfully so—obliterating the intimacy intended by God. Without due care, this intrusion can have permanent aftereffects, not only for the relationship of the couple, but for the child as well.

In the context of discipleship, Jesus warns us to count the cost, a warning that is applicable to the use of reproductive technologies as well. Costs must be carefully weighed, for they are neither insubstantial nor insignificant. In our culture, we understand technology to be a great good and we take its use for granted, assuming that if it is available it should certainly be used. We need to explore what we believe about family, children, sexuality, and God, prayerfully reflecting on these issues in light of Scripture. We can then move ahead in God's grace, trusting Him to provide abundantly for the desires of our hearts as He sees fit and in His time.

As an obstetrician-gynecologist who has cared for infertility patients for many years, walking with them through the struggles, the sorrows, and the joys, I applaud Scott and Joy's work, for they have navigated these complexities with skill and compassion.

**SUSAN M. HAACK,** *MD, FACOG, MA Bioethics*
*Friendship, Wisconsin*

# Notes

## Chapter 1: The Experience of Infertility

1. Stepping Stones publishes a regular newsletter; their web address is: http://www.bethany.org/step.

2. The CDC defines ART according to the 1992 Fertility Clinic Success Rate and Certification Act.

3. To be exact, GIFT, ZIFT, and IVF normally involve the genetic materials of husband and wife only, though they can be used with donor genetic materials too. For egg donation to work, one of the above techniques must also be employed.

4. See chapter 3 for a more extended discussion of the Roman Catholic contribution to reproductive ethics.

5. http://www.cdc.gov/nchs/fastats/fertile.htm; page last updated April 2, 2009.

6. "Infertility: An Overview," *American Society for Reproductive Medicine* (2003): 7–12.

7. Department of Health and Human Services, Centers for Disease Control and Prevention, "Infertility: A Public Health Focus on Infertility Prevention, Detection, and Management," http://www.cdc.gov/reproductivehealth/Infertility/Whitepaper-PG1.htm.

8. International Committee for Monitoring Assisted Reproductive Technology (IC-MART), World Collaborative Report on Assisted Reproductive Technology, 2002, *Human Reproduction* 24 (2009): 2310–20.

9. Clinic Summary Report, 2008, All Treatment Types, https://www.sartcorsonline.com/rptCSR_PublicMultYear.aspx?ClinicPKID=0.

10. Debra L. Spar, *The Baby Business: How Money, Science, and Politics Drive the Commerce of Conception* (Boston: Harvard Business School Publishing Corporation, 2006), table 1-1, 3.

11. Department of Health and Human Services, Centers for Disease Control and Prevention, "Infertility: A Public Health Focus on Infertility Prevention, Detection, and Management," http://www.cdc.gov/http://www.cdc.gov/reproductivehealth/Infertility/Whitepaper-PG1.htm.

12. Spar, 5.

## Chapter 2: Theology of Family and Procreation

1. Works that include the discussion (some very brief) of technologically assisted procreation are Andreas Kostenberger, *God, Marriage and the Family* (Wheaton: Crossway, 2004), 129–51; Dennis P. Hollinger, *The Meaning of Sex* (Grand Rapids: Baker Academic, 2009),199–222; Stanley J. Grenz, *Sexual Ethics* (Louisville: Westminster John Knox, 1990), 163–77; David VanDrunen, *Bioethics and the Christian Life* (Wheaton: Crossway, 2009), 119–45; Sandra L. Glahn and William R. Cutrer, *The Infertility Companion* (Grand Rapids: Zondervan, 2004), 145–218; H. Tristam Englehardt Jr., *The Foundations of Christian Bioethics* (Lisse, Netherlands: Swets & Zeitlinger, 2000), 233–308; Allen Verhey, *Reading the Bible in the Strange World of Medicine* (Grand Rapids: Eerdmans, 2003), 253-303; Brent Waters, *Reproductive Technology: Toward a Theology of Procreative Stewardship* (Cleveland: The Pilgrim Press, 2001); Oliver O'Donovan, *Begotten or Made?* (Oxford: Clarendon Press, 1984); Ted Peters, *For the Love of Children* (Louisville: Westminster John Knox Press, 1996), 119–82.

2. Walter C. Kaiser Jr., *Toward Old Testament Ethics* (Grand Rapids: Zondervan, 1983), 153–54. See also Gordon J. Wenham, *Genesis 1–15*, Word Biblical Commentary, vol. 1 (Nashville: Thomas Nelson, 1987), 71; and Allen P. Ross, *Creation and Blessing: A Guide to the Study and Exposition of the Book of Genesis* (Grand Rapids: Baker, 1988).

3. Some scholars insist that the "leaving" is more emotional and psychological than geographic and physical, since the tradition of extended families was so strong in the ancient world. We would suggest that the husband-wife-children unit was basic to the family regardless of how extended it became due to economic and cultural reasons. See Gordon J. Wenham, "Family in the Pentateuch," in Richard S. Hess and M. Daniel Carroll R., eds., *Family in the Bible: Exploring Customs, Culture and Context* (Grand Rapids: Baker, 2003), 17–18.

4. Other purposes for sex include pleasure (Song of Solomon; Prov. 5:15–20) and the establishment of oneness between the married couple (Gen. 2:25; 1 Cor. 6:16). See the discussion of this in Dennis Hollinger, *The Meaning of Sex: Christian Ethics and the Moral Life* (Grand Rapids: Baker, 2009), 93–115. We would also argue that marriage has multiple ends, but procreation is a unique end of marriage.

5. Christopher J. H. Wright, *Old Testament Ethics for the People of God* (Downers Grove: InterVarsity Press, 2004), 330.

6. Brent Waters, *Reproductive Technology: Toward a Theology of Procreative Stewardship* (Cleveland: The Pilgrim Press, 2001), 52–53.

7. Ibid., 83.

8. Norman L. Geisler, *Christian Ethics* (Grand Rapids, Zondervan, 1990), 187. See also Sandra L. Glahn and William R. Cutrer, *The Infertility Companion* (Grand Rapids: Zondervan, 2004), 187–88, who do end up qualifying their view somewhat.

9. Oliver O'Donovan, *Begotten or Made?* (Oxford: Clarendon Press, 1984), 42–44.

10. Christopher J. H. Wright insists that monogamy was the more common practice of the majority of the population, and OT examples of polygamy are those of kings or those in leadership positions of some prestige. See Wright, *Old Testament Ethics for the People of God*, 330.

11. John H. Walton and Victor H. Matthews, *The IVP Bible Background Commentary: Genesis–Deuteronomy* (Grand Rapids: Zondervan, 1997), 23.

12. Ibid., 42.

13. I am indebted to my colleague Dr. Ken Way for his description of the law as a means of "damage control" in a fallen world.

14. O'Donovan, 40.

## Chapter 3: Catholic Natural Law and Procreation

1. Not only do the official Catholic encyclicals address reproductive technology, but so do numerous Catholic moral theologians. For example, until very recently, when my students ask me for theologically oriented resources that deal with reproductive technologies, all I was able to recommend were sources by Roman Catholic authors. My experience is likely the norm for evangelicals interested in bioethics. Evangelical sources that did exist at all were few, and they were frequently on the simplistic side, either in affirmation or dissent. See for example, Donald DeMarco, *Biotechnology and the Assault on Parenthood* (San Francisco: Ignatius Press, 1991); Jérôme Lejeune, *The Concentration Can: When Does Human Life Begin?* (San Francisco: Ignatius Press, 1992). Dissenting voices (in varying degrees of dissent) include Charles E. Curran and Julie Hanlon Rubio, eds., *Marriage Readings in Moral Theology*, Vol. 15 (New York: Paulist Press, 2009); Lisa Sowle Cahill *Theological Bioethics: Participation, Justice, and Change* (Washington, D.C.: Georgetown University Press, 2005).

2. For further information on Catholic teaching in this area, see Edward Collins Vacek, S.J., "Catholic 'Natural Law' and Reproductive Ethics," *Journal of Medicine & Philosophy* 17 (1992): 329–46. His work will be referred to later in this chapter.

3. Paul VI, Encyc. *Humanae Vitae*, July 28, 1968, paragraph 9. The encyclical was published in English in A.A.S. IX (September 30, 1969), no. 9: 481–518. This citation is taken from page 486.

4. Ibid., paragraph 12, 488.

5. Ibid., paragraph 13, 489.

6. This document is published in *Origins* 16, no. 40 (March 19, 1987): 698–710.

7. Ibid., 699–700.

8. Ibid., 700.

9. "Instruction," 704–5.

10. The Instruction uses the term "heterologous artificial fertilization" to describe these. For technologies that use the genetic material of husband and wife, the Instruction terms these "homologous artificial fertilization."

11. Ibid., 705.

12. Ibid.

13. Ibid., 706.

14. Ibid.

15. Ibid., 707.

16. Ibid.

17. Benedict XVI, Instruction *Dignitas Personae* On Certain Bioethical Questions, June 20, 2008, http://www.vatican.va/roman_curia/congregations/cfaith/documents/rc_con_cfaith_doc_20081208_dignitas-personae_en.html.

18. Richard A. McCormick, S.J., "Therapy or Tampering?: The Ethics of Reproductive Technology," *America* 154 (December 7, 1985), cited in Arthur L. Greil, "The Religious Response to Reproductive Technology," *The Christian Century* (January 4–11, 1989): 11–14, at 12.

19. Instruction, 708.

20. Vacek, "Catholic Natural Law and Reproductive Ethics," 338.

21. Ibid.

22. Sidney Callahan, "Lovemaking and Babymaking," *Commonweal* 114 (1987): 233–39, at 234.

23. For discussion of the parameters of the direct use of these techniques, see chapters 5 (for artificial insemination) and 6 (for in vitro fertilization, GIFT, and ZIFT).

## Chapter 4: The Moral Status of Fetuses and Embryos

1. Such dominion involves the freedom to use creation for mankind's benefit, but man was also given responsibility for creation as God's steward. This responsibility prevents mankind from exploiting the environment under the guise of dominion over it. See Genesis 1:28–29.

2. For further discussion of the incarnation of Jesus and its relevance to the moral status of the unborn, see David Atkinson, "Some Theological Perspectives on the Human Embryo," in Nigel M. De S. Cameron, ed., *Embryos and Ethics: The Warnock Report in Debate* (Edinburgh: Rutherford House Books, 1987), 54–55.

3. For more on this text, see Umberto Cassuto, *Exodus* (Jerusalem: Magnes Press, 1967), 275; and Gleason Archer, *Encyclopedia of Bible Difficulties* (Grand Rapids: Zondervan, 1982), 246–49.

4. cf. Richard Werner, "Abortion: The Moral status of the Unborn," *Social Theory and Practice,* vol. 4 (spring 1975): 201–22.

5. See for example, Bonnie Steinbock, *Life Before Birth: The Moral and Legal Status of Embryos and Fetuses* (New York: Oxford University Press, 1996).

6. There is some debate on the parallel between killing and allowing to die in euthanasia. See for example, James Rachels, *The End of Life* (New York: Oxford University Press, 1987).

7. For examples of those who articulate this view, see Steinbock, 59–61; Laurence Tribe, *Abortion: The Clash of Absolutes* (New York: W. W. Norton, 1990), 234–35; and Peter Singer and Karen Dawson, "IVF Technology and the Argument from Potential," in Peter Singer et al., eds., *Embryo Experimentation: Ethical, Legal and Social Issues* (Cambridge: Cambridge University Press, 1990), 76–77.

8. Robert P. George and Christopher Tollefsen, *Embryo: A Defense of Human Life* (New York: Doubleday, 2008), 51.

9. For more on this see J. P. Moreland and Scott B. Rae, *Body & Soul: Human Nature & the Crisis in Ethics* (Downers Grove, IL: IVP Academic, 2000), 271–74.

10. George J. Annas, "A French Homonculus in a Tennessee Court," *Hastings Center Report* 19 (November–December 1989): 22.

11. Moral philosopher James Rachels popularized this distinction, more specifically with regard to the debate over assisted suicide and euthanasia. See Rachels, *The End of Life* (New York: Oxford Press, 1987).

12. Mary Ann Warren, "On the Moral and Legal Status of Abortion," James P. Sterba, ed., *Morality in Practice* (Hartford: Wadsworth, 2003), 144–45. Quoted by W. F. Cooney, "The Fallacy of All Person-Denying Arguments for Abortion," *Journal of Applied Philosophy* 8, no.2 (1991): 163. See also Mary Anne Warren, *Moral Status: Obligations to Persons and Other Living Things* (New York: Oxford University Press, 1997).

13. Joseph Fletcher, "Indicators of Humanhood: A Tentative Profile," *Hastings Center Report* vol. 2 (1972). Cited by Scott B. Rae, "Views of Human Nature at the Edges of Life," J. P. Moreland and David Ciocchi, eds., *Christian Perspectives on Being Human: A Multidisciplinary Approach to Integration* (Grand Rapids: Baker, 1993), 239.

14. This is helpfully stated by Patrick Lee in *Abortion and Unborn Human Life* (Washington, D.C.: Catholic University of America Press, 1996).

15. Ibid., 260.

16. Helga Kuhse and Peter Singer, *Should the Baby Live?* (New York: Oxford Press, 1985), 133. It is quickly apparent that Kuhse and Singer equivocate on the question of personal identity. After all, if I do not exist until sometime after my birth, in what sense is the birth mine? The only way for "*my* birth" to be more than a linguistic convention is to admit that "I" existed before I was born, or at least at the time of my birth. But if this is the case, Kuhse and Singer's attempt to define personhood in terms of function fails.

## Chapter 5: Intrauterine Insemination and Egg Donation

1. See the discussion of GIFT, ZIFT, and IVF for examples of technologies that are generally allowed but with restrictions.

2. "Medicine: Artificial Bastards?" *Time*, Monday, Feb. 26, 1945, http://www.time.com/time/magazine/article/0,9171,792012,00.html.

3. Bruce L. Wilder, "Assisted Reproduction Technology: Trends and Suggestions for the Developing Law," *Assisted Reproduction Technology*, vol. 18, 2002: 177.

4. "Artificial Insemination: Practice in the United States: Summary of a 1987 Survey" (August 1988), http://www.princeton.edu/~ota/ns20/alpha_f.html.

5. David Plotz, *The Genius Factory* (New York: Random House Trade Paperbacks, 2006; Random House, 2005), 170.

6. See website of the California Cryobank at https://www.spermbank.com/cd_secure/newdonors/index.cfm.

7. California Cryobank, "Donor—Extensive Search Criteria," http://www.cryobank.com/Donor-Search/Advanced-Search.

8. Fairfax Cryobank, "Donor Search," http://donorsearch.fairfaxcryobank.com.

9. American Society for Reproductive Medicine, Third Party Reproduction, *A Guide for Patients (Sperm, egg, and embryo donation and surrogacy)*, http://asrm.org/publications/index.aspx?id=76.

10. Rainbow Flag Sperm Bank, information available at http://www.gayspermbank.com/index.html.

11. Lisa Jean Moore, *Sperm Counts: Overcome by Man's Most Precious Fluid* (New York: NYU Press, 2007), 104, table 1.

12. Many sperm banks do not show a dollar amount, but at least one shows a range:http://ny.cryosinternational.com/become-a-donor/donor-information. aspx. One sperm bank shows a payment of $500 per donation for "open donor" sperm: http://www.sperm1.com/sbny/donor.html#Anchor-How-49575.

13. Rachel Lehmann-Haupt, "Mapping the God of Sperm," *Newsweek*, December 16, 2009, http://www.newsweek.com/id/227104/page/1.

14. See Gina Kolata, "Young Women Offer to Sell Their Eggs to Infertile Couples," *New York Times* (November 19, 1991); and Robin Herman, "Egg Donation Centers More Accessible Today," *Washington Post* (July 14, 1992), cited in Andrew Kimbrell, *The Human Body Shop* (New York: Harper Collins, 1993), 83.

15. "2006 Assisted Reproductive Technology (ART) Report: Section 1—Overview," http://www.cdc.gov/ART/ART2006/section1.htm#f2.

16. Moore, *Sperm Counts,* 104, table 1.

17. Aaron D. Levine, "Self-Regulation, Compensation, and the Ethical Recruitment of Oocyte Donors," *Hastings Center Report* 40, no 2 (2010): 25–36. Read more: http://www.thehastingscenter.org/Publications/HCR/Detail. aspx?id=4549#ixzz0jgY9zzMx.

18. Julia Derek, *Confessions of a Serial Egg Donor* (New York: Adrenaline Books, 2004), back cover.

19. Moore, *Sperm Counts,* 104, table 1.

20. Uniform Parentage Act, section 5 (b).

21. In some cases, there might be medical reasons for reducing the number of pregnancies a woman is carrying, but those cases are rare. For further discussion of selective termination, see chapter 6.

22. Kirsty Horsey, "European Parliament Calls for Egg Trade Ban," *Progress Educational Trust,* March 16, 2005, http://www.ivf.net/ivf/european_parliament_calls_for_egg_trade_ban-o1326.html.

23. Katrina George, "Women Overlooked in Biotech Debate, Human Cloning Exploitive," August 22, 2006, http://www.lifenews.com/bio1725.html.

24. Helen Pearson, "Health Effects of Egg Donation May Take Decades to Emerge," *Nature* 442, 607–8 (August 10, 2006), doi:10.1038/442607a; Published online August 9, 2006, http://www.nature.com/nature/journal/v442/n7103/full/442607a.html.

25. See David Blankenhorn, *Fatherless America* (New York: Harper Perennial, 1996).

26. Kristina Fiore, "Births Outside Marriage on the Rise," MedPage, May 13, 2009, http://www.medpagetoday.com/OBGYN/Pregnancy/14195?userid=119821&impressionId=1242268518210&utm_source=mSpoke&utm_medium=email&utm_campaign=DailyHeadlines&utm_content=Group1.

27. John Leo, "Promoting No-Dad Families," *U.S. News and World* Report, May 15, 1995, 26.

28. Daniel Callahan, "Bioethics and Fatherhood," *Utah Law Review* 1992:3 (1992): 735–46.

29. Nick Pisa, "Britain's oldest mum-to-be warned 66 is too old—by Rosanna Della Corte, mum at 63," *Mirror.co.uk.news*, August 18, 2009, http://www.mirror.co.uk/news/top-stories/2009/05/18/britain-s-oldest-mum-to-be-warned-66-is-too-old-by-rosanna-della-corte-mum-at-63-115875-21367784/.

30. Ibid.

31. William D. Montalbano, "Physicians Ban Controversial Biogenetics," *Los Angeles Times*, April 15, 1995, A2.

32. Tina Molly Lang "Britain's Elizabeth Munro Pregnant at 66," *Associated Content*, May 18, 2009, http://www.associatedcontent.com/article/1758986/britains_elizabeth_munro_pregnant_at.html.

33. Sheryl Stolberg, "Science Helps Italian Woman Give Birth at 62," *Los Angeles Times*, July 19, 1994, A2.

34. Plotz, 57.

35. http://www.donorsiblingregistry.com/.

36. Plotz, 82.

37. Katrina Clark, "My Father Was an Anonymous Sperm Donor," *Washington Post,* Sunday, December 17, 2006, http://www.washingtonpost.com/wp-dyn/content/article/2006/12/15/AR2006121501820.html.

## Chapter 6: GIFT, ZIFT, and IVF

1. The Centers for Disease Control and Prevention is responsible for the collection and reporting of live birth rates of ART clinics in the United States. This is in accordance with the Fertility Clinic Success Rate and Certification Act of 1992. The American Society for Reproductive Medicine (ASRM) website directs readers to the CDC: "All Assisted Reproductive Technology Success Rates National Summary and Fertility Clinic Reports can be viewed at the CDC Internet site at: http://www.cdc.gov/ART/index.htm." Available at http://www.asrm.org/news/article.aspx?id=409.

2. One of the more helpful portions of the CDC site includes this document: "How to Read a Fertility Clinic Table," http://www.cdc.gov/ART/ART2006/htrfct.htm.

3. Cycles reported here include for women up to age forty-two for both fresh embryos from nondonor eggs and frozen embryos from nondonor eggs. CDC, "Assisted Reproductive Technology (ART) Report: National Summary," http://apps.nccd.cdc.gov/art/.

4. Some clinics do not offer selective termination to their clients, but may refer to a physician who does offer it.

5. In some states, such as California, state law requires insurance companies to offer coverage for assisted reproduction. It may that in some states the premium is so high that it discourages people from buying the coverage, or it may only cover a relatively small percentage of the costs. However, many insurance companies do offer such coverage at a reasonable cost. According to the Society for Human Resource Management, 23 percent of employee benefits in 2009 included coverage for in vitro fertilization, but to what extent IVF was covered is not detailed. http://www.shrm.org/Research/SurveyFindings/Articles/Documents/09-0295_Emp_Benefits_SR_Tables.pdf. To what extent ART will be covered (if any) by the 2010 Patient Protection and Affordable Care Act is unclear currently.

6. In Italy, no more than three embryos may be produced, and all must be implanted at the same time (with rare exception). Andrea Boggio, "Italy enacts new law on medically assisted reproduction," published by Oxford University Press on behalf of the European Society of Human Reproduction and Embryology, March 24, 2005, http://humrep.oxfordjournals.org/cgi/reprint/deh871v1.pdf, page 2 of five. Germany has a similar law, per "Germany's embryo protection law is 'killing embryos rather than protecting them,'" ESHRE Press Release, July 5, 2007, http://www.ivf.net/ivf/germany_s_embryo_protection_law_is_killing_embryos_rather_than_protecting_them-o2806.html.

7. "How Many Frozen Human Embryos Are Available for Research?" Rand Law & Health Research Brief, http://www.rand.org/pubs/research_briefs/RB9038/index1.html.

8. Fran Lowry, "Guidelines Updated on Number of Embryos to Be Transferred During In Vitro Fertilization," *Medscape Internal Medicine* from WebMD, http://www.medscape.com/viewarticle/710965.

9. See the discussion of the personhood of the fetus/embryo in chapter 4 for more detail on this concept.

10. "Q7: Does In Vitro Fertilization Work?" American Society for Reproductive Medicine, http://www.asrm.org/detail.aspx?id=3024.

11. "How Many Frozen Human Embryos Are Available for Research?" http://www.rand.org/pubs/research_briefs/RB9038/index1.html.

12. Daniel Schorn, "A Surplus of Embryos: What Should Happen with Extra Embryos?" *CBS 60 Minutes*, reported by Leslie Stahl, February 12, 2006, http://www.cbsnews.com/stories/2006/02/09/60minutes/main1300667.shtml?tag=contentMain;contentBody.

13. The Ethics Committee of the American Society for Reproductive Medicine, "Disposition of abandoned embryos," *Fertility and Sterility,* 82, suppl. 1 (September 2004): S253, http://www.asrm.org/topics/detail.aspx?id=408; "abandonedembryos-1.pdf".

14. Roger Rosenblatt, *Time* (February 14, 1983): 90.

15. For more detail on this case, see George P. Smith, "Australia's Frozen 'Orphan' Embryos: A Medical, Legal and Ethical Dilemma," *Journal of Family Law* 24:1 (1985–86): 26-41. See also Donald DeMarco, *Biotechnology and the Assault on Parenthood* (San Francisco: Ignatius Press, 1991): 104–5.

16. Davis v. Davis, 1990 Tenn. App. LEXIS 642 (September 13, 1990).

17. For further reading on the Davis case, see George J. Annas, "Crazy-Making: Embryos and Gestational Mothers," *Hastings Center Report* 21 (January–February 1991): 35–38; and Alexander Morgan Capron, "Parenthood and Frozen Embryos: More than Property and Privacy," *Hastings Center Report* 22 (September–October 1992): 32–33.

18. Tao Tao and Alfonso Del Valle "Human oocyte and ovarian tissue cryopreservation and its application," *Journal of Assisted Reproductive Genetics* 25 (July 2008): 287–96. Published online 2008 August 1. doi: 10.1007/ s10815-008-9236-z, http://www.ncbi.nlm.nih.gov/pmc/articles/ PMC2596676/?tool=pubmed.

19. Of course, the legal system would view these differently. More direct killing would surely receive a harsher sentence. Allowing someone to die might carry a manslaughter charge. It is true that most states do not have Good Samaritan laws that require people to render aid to someone who is in trouble (physicians are excepted from this and are required). But most would agree that allowing someone to die when you could have easily prevented his or her death is morally reprehensible.

20. For further reading on this view, see Francis J. Beckwith, *Defending Life: A Moral and Legal Case against Abortion Choice* (New York: Cambridge University Press, 2007): 65–92.

21. Human ova (eggs) are in great demand for use by the fertility industry as well as for research. The prospect of discarding human eggs when so much could be done seemingly "for good" seems unlikely to the authors. So, while egg freezing may solve one problem, it may create a number of others, seen and unforeseen.

22. Letitia Stein, "Sarasota doctor loses medical license for aborting wrong fetus," http://www.tampabay.com/news/health/sarasota-doctor-loses-medical-license-for-aborting-wrong-fetus/1086967, Tampabay.com, April 13, 2010.

23. Ibid.

24. Data from 2003, https://www.sartcorsonline.com/rptCSR_PublicMultYear. aspx?ClinicPKID=0.

25. Rachel Gurevich, ICSI—Intracytoplasmic Sperm Injection: What you need to know about ICSI, updated July 6, 2009, http://infertility.about.com/od/ivf/a/ icsi_ivf.htm.

26. K. Wisborg, H. J. Ingerslev, and T. B. Henriksen, "IVF and stillbirth: a prospective follow-up study," http://humrep.oxfordjournals.org.

27. U. B. Wennerholm, et al, "Incidence of congenital malformations in children born after ICSI," http://humrep.oxfordjournals.org/cgi/content/full/15/4/94 4?view=long&pmid=10739847.

28. "Increased prevalence of imprinting defects in patients with Angelman syndrome born to subfertile couples," *Journal of Medical Genetics* 42 (2005): 289–91, http://jmg.bmj.com/content/42/4/289.long.

29. "Beckwith-Wiedemann syndrome and assisted reproduction technology (ART)," *Journal of Medical Genetics* 40 (2003): 62–64, http://jmg.bmj.com/content/40/1/62.long.

## Chapter 7: Surrogate Motherhood

1. For further discussion of this case, see In re Buzzanca, 72 Cal. Rptr. 2d at 282; see also Christen Blackburn, "Who Is a Mother? Determining Legal Maternity in Surrogacy Arrangements in Tennessee," 39 University of Memphis Law Review (2009): 349–81, at 354–56.

2. In the matter of Baby M, 537 A. 2d, 1249 (1988).

3. Johnson v. Calvert (851 P.2d 776, 1993).

4. In the matter of Baby M, Ibid.

5. This real estate analogy is taken from Alexander M. Capron, "Surrogate Contracts: A Danger Zone," *Los Angeles Times*, April 7, 1987, B5.

6. For more on the globalization of surrogacy, see Susan Markens, *Surrogate Motherhood and the Politics of Reproduction* (Berkeley: University of California Press, 2007), 4–9; Usha Rengachary Smerdon, "Crossing Bodies, Crossing Borders: International Surrogacy Between the United States and India," 39 *Cumberland Law Review* (2008): 15–83; Ruby L. Lee, "New Trends in Global Outsourcing of Commercial Surrogacy: A Call for Regulation," 20 *Hastings Women's Law Journal* (2008): 275–300.

7. Statement of staff psychologist Howard Adelman of Surrogate Mothering Ltd. in Philadelphia, cited in Gena Corea, *The Mother Machine* (New York: Harper and Row, 1985), 229.

8. Krittivas Mukherjee, "Rent-a-womb in India fuels surrogate motherhood debate," *Reuters*, February 5, 2007, http://www.reuters.com/article/idUSDEL 29873520070205.

9. Cited in Gena Corea, *The Mother Machine* (New York: Harper and Row, 1985), 245.

10. Cited in Corea, 214–15. For discussion of some of the legal protections advised to prevent such exploitation, see Jennifer Rimm, "Booming Baby Business: Regulating Commercial Surrogacy in India," 30 University of Pennsylvania Journal of International Law (2009): 1429–62.

11. This sounds worse than it may be since Mary Beth Whitehead had left the area with the child because she wanted so badly to keep her. The police were obeying the dictates of a lower court decision that awarded sole custody of the child to the contracting couple. But in any case, they still took the child by force from the woman who bore her. That struck most people as unfortunate if not barbaric.

12. In Stanley v. Illinois, the Supreme Court stated that "the rights to conceive and to raise one's children have been deemed essential . . . basic civil rights of man . . . , far more precious than property rights. It is cardinal with us that the custody, care and nurture of the child reside first in the parents." 405 U.S. 650 (1971), at 651.

13. Arthur Martin, "Baby number 8 on the way for the mother of all surrogates," *MailOnline*, January 6, 2010, http://www.dailymail.co.uk/news/article-1240870/Baby-No-8-way-mother-surrogates.html#ixzz0oPJlHC2j.

14. Denis Campbell, "Couples who pay surrogate mothers could lose right to raise the child," *The Guardian*, April 5, 2010, http://www.guardian.co.uk/uk/2010/apr/05/surrogacy-parents-ivf.

15. Daniel Callahan, "Surrogate Motherhood: A Bad Idea," *New York Times*, January 20, 1987, B21.

16. Katharine T. Bartlett, "Re-expressing parenthood," *Yale Law Journal* 98 (1988): 333–34.

17. See for example, Andrea Stumpf, "Redefining Mother: A Legal Matrix for New Reproductive Technologies," *Yale Law Review* 96 (1986): 197–208; Marjorie Maguire Schultz, "Reproductive Technology and Intent-Based Parenthood: An Opportunity for Gender Neutrality," *Wisconsin Law Review* 2 (1990): 298–398.

18. ACOG Committee on Ethics, Committee Opinion No. 397, "Surrogate Motherhood," American College of Obstetricians and Gynecologists. *Obstet Gynecol* 2008; 111:465–70, http://www.acog.org/from_home/publications/ethics/co397.pdf.

19. United Kingdom, Department of Health and Social Security.1984. Report of the Committee of Inquiry into Human Fertilization and Embryology. Cited in Edgar Page, "Donation, Surrogacy and Adoption," *Journal of Applied Philosophy* 2 (1985): 162.

20. Ruth Macklin, "Artificial Means of Reproduction and Our Understanding of the Family," *Hastings Center Report* 21 (January–February 1991): 9. See also Amy M. Larkey, "Redefining Motherhood: Determining Legal Maternity in Gestational Surrogacy Arrangements," *Drake Law Review* 51 (2003): 605–32.

21. See note, "Rumpelstiltskin Revisited: The Inalienable Rights of Surrogate Mothers," *Harvard Law Review* 99 (June 1986): 1952.

22. Barbara Davies, "Billion-dollar baby trade: The darker side of adoption," *Mail Online*, November 2, 2007, http://www.dailymail.co.uk/femail/article-491440/Billion-dollar-baby-trade-The-darker-adoption.html#ixzz0oPZpz0V0.

23. This is discussed further in Christen Blackburn, "Who Is a Mother? Determining Legal Maternity in Surrogacy Arrangements in Tennessee," *University of Memphis Law Review* 39 (2009): 349–82.

24. Macklin, "Artificial Means of Reproduction and Our Understanding of the Family," 9.

25. The Donor Sibling Registry is available at www.donorsiblingregistry.com.

26. See Macklin, 9. The concept of gametes, and the parental rights that accompany them, being transferable is taken from Edgar Page, "Donation, Surrogacy and Adoption," 165.

27. Johnson v. Calvert, Supreme Court of the State of California, SO23721, May 20, 1993, 13.

28. For further discussion of this view, see John New, "Aren't You Lucky You Have Two Mamas?: Redefining Parenthood in Light of Evolving Reproductive Technologies and Social Change," 81 *Chicago-Kent Law Review* (2006): 773–808.

## Chapter 8: Prenatal Genetic Testing

1. Dr. Henderson, as well as the patients described, while representative of others who have similar life journeys are totally fictitious, and do not represent any particular person(s) known to the authors.

2. "Update on Carrier Screening for Cystic Fibrosis." ACOG Committee Opinion No. 325, American College of Obstetricians and Gynecologists. Obstet Gynecol 2005; 106: 1465–68.

3. For more information, see www.mayoclinic.com/health/medical/IM04422.

4. Interview by author, D. Joy Riley, Smyrna, Tennessee, May 25, 2010. For additional information, see www.mayoclinic.com/health/amniocentesis/MY0115.

5. For further information, see L. P. Shulman and S. Elias, "Amniocentesis and Chorionic Villas Sampling," Western Journal of Medicine, September 1993: 159 (3): 260–68. Available at www.ncbi.nlm.nih.gov/pmc/articles/pmc10113381/?page=7.

6. Interview by author D. Joy Riley, Smyrna, Tennessee, May 15, 2010. For additional information, see www.webmd.com/baby/guide/prenatal-tests.

7. Philip Hunter, "Preimplantation Genetic Diagnosis"—The Scientist—Magazine of the Life Sciences, http://www.the-scientist.com/article/display/14771/#ixzz0rRnaQA7B.

8. Genetics and Public Policy Center, "Publication announcement—Preimplantation genetic screening: a survey of in vitro fertilization clinics," http://www.dnapolicy.org/news.enews.article.nocategory.php?action=detail&newsletter_id=36&article_id=163.

9. For further information on the project at a more popular level, see Robert Sha-piro, *The Human Blueprint* (New York: St. Martin's Press, 1991); and Lois Wing-erson, *Mapping Our Genes* (New York: Plume Books, 1990). For a more academic view, see George J. Annas and Sherman Elias, *Gene Mapping: Using Law and Ethics as Guides* (New York: Oxford University Press, 1992).

10. Francis S. Collins, "A Brief Primer on Genetic Testing," http://www.genome. gov/10506784.

11. NCBI, "Gene Tests," http://www.ncbi.nlm.nih.gov/sites GeneTests/ ?db=GeneTests.

12. That is not to say that any specific genetic disease is the result of a specific sin committed by one of the parents of the child in question—far from it. Genetic diseases are the result of the general presence of sin in the world.

13. Even the scholarly literature on the subject makes this presumption. For exam-ple, Kathleen Nolan, M.D., an associate of the Hastings Center, states that, "Out of respect for reproductive decision making and genetic privacy, and to prevent abuses such as attempts at eugenic control, virtually all genetic counselors espouse the ideals of value-neutral counseling and autonomous decision mak-ing." "First Fruits: Genetic Screening," in "Genetic Grammar: Health, Illness and the Human Genome Project," Special Supplement, *Hastings Center Report* 22 (July–August 1992): S2–4.

14. Though also lamenting the loss of choice for parents who desire to raise a handicapped child, sociologist Barbara Katz Rothman nevertheless makes this assumption too when she states that, "Although some people have discussed the value of being forewarned of genetic or other diseases even in a pregnancy the woman intends to carry to term, abortion is an integral part of this new technol-ogy [of prenatal testing]" in "The Products of Conception: The Social Context of Reproductive Choices," *Journal of Medical Ethics* 11 (1985): 188–192, at 189.

15. Elizabeth Kristol, "Picture Perfect: The Politics of Prenatal Testing," *First Things* (April 1993), 18, 20.

16. Francis J. Beckwith, *Defending Life: A Moral and Legal Case against Abortion Choice* (New York: Cambridge University Press, 2007).

17. Some time ago I overheard a nurse discussing the care of anencephalic child. The parents were trying to decide how much treatment to authorize, and the nurse suggested that "this decision is easy. Take the child home and let it die. It's not a person."

18. For further discussion of this aspect of personhood see the material in chapter 4. See also Scott B. Rae, "Views of Human Nature at the Edges of Life: Person-hood and Medical Ethics," in J. P. Moreland and David M. Ciocchi eds., *Christian Perspectives on Being Human: A Multidisciplinary Approach to Integration* (Grand Rapids: Baker Book House, 1993), 235–56. See also J.P. Moreland and Scott B. Rae, *Body and Soul: Human Nature and the Crisis in Ethics* (Downers Grove, IL: IVP Academic, 2000).

19. For more detail on this voluminous debate see, J.P. Moreland, "James Rachels and the Active Euthanasia Debate," *Journal of the Evangelical Theological Society* 31 (March 1988): 81–94, and idem. "Review of the End of Life," *The Thomist* 53 (October 1989): 714–22.

20. Philip Hunter, in "Preimplantation Genetic Diagnosis"—The Scientist—Magazine of the Life Sciences, http://www.thescientist.com/article/display/14771/.

21. Even though the NIH panel for embryo research recognized that special moral status should be granted to the embryo, they and many others do not see embryos on the same moral level with fetuses. For example, Professor Andrea Bonnicksen states that, "Arguably it is morally more acceptable to discard embryos than to abort fetuses." She further adds that, "Deliberately discarding faulty embryos is arguably no worse than the constant threat in IVF of embryo loss due to biological fluke." In the first statement, she apparently assumes that implantation makes a morally significant difference in determining personhood, but that is only a difference in location, not essence. In this second statement, she ignores the obvious difference between accidental death of embryos and intentional discarding of defective embryos. "Genetic Diagnosis of Human Embryos," *Hastings Center Report*, 22 Special Supplement (July–August 1992): S5–11, at 5–6.

22. Genetics and IVF Institute, MicroSort. Available at http://microsort.net/index.php.

23. See for example, Wendy Rogers, Angela Ballantyne, and Heather Draper, "Is Sex-Selective Abortion Morally Justified and Should It Be Prohibited?" *Bioethics* 21:9 (2007): 520–24. For a contrasting view, see Edgar Dahl, "Procreative Liberty: The Case for Preconception Sex Selection," *Reproductive BioMedicine OnLine* 7:4 (October–November 2003): 380–84.

24. Jane Macartney, "China tries to sterilise 10,000 parents over one-child rule," *Times Online*, April 17, 2010, http://www.timesonline.co.uk/tol/news/world/asia/article7099417.ece.

25. "Chinese gender imbalance will leave millions of men without wives," *Telegraph.co.uk*, January 11, 2010, http://www.telegraph.co.uk/news/worldnews/asia/china/6966037/Chinese-gender-imbalance-will-leave-millions-of-men-without-wives.html.

26. For discussion of this, see Shanam Saini, "Born *TO DIE*," *Humanist* 62:4 (Jul/Aug 2002): 25–28; Steven W. Mosher, "China's One-Child Policy: Twenty-five Years Later," *Human Life Review* 32:1 (winter 2006): 76–101.

27. "Chinese Gender Imbalance," 1.

28. Ibid.

29. Kristol, 23.

30. Cited in Kristol, 23.

31. Rothman, "The Products of Conception," 190.

# Acknowledgments

I (Scott) want to express my gratitude to a variety of people who were instrumental in getting this project to become a reality. Thanks to Madison Trammel at Moody Publishers, who approached me some time ago with the idea of doing this book, and in a partnership with Dr. Riley. I'm very grateful to Dr. Riley for her contribution to this book and for being such a delight to work with. Thanks to our editor, Pam Pugh, who took our joint work and made it sound like a single person—thanks for your careful and thorough work to make this read far better than we could ourselves. Special thanks go to my research assistant, Jessica Mefford, who compiled and summarized much of the material that went into the various sidebars throughout the book. I'm also grateful to my deans at Talbot School of Theology, Biola University, Dr. Dennis Dirks and Dr. Mike Wilkins, for the sabbatical leave in the spring of 2010 that enabled me to devote myself to this project. I so appreciate the encouragement of my colleagues in the department of philosophy at Talbot—it is a joy to work with you guys and to have your support for my research and writing. And special thanks to my family, my wife, Sally, and sons Taylor, Cameron, and Austin: I appreciate your patience as I worked to get this finished. You guys are the best!

(Joy) There are many who have helped and supported my contribution to this project. I am grateful for Scott Rae, who welcomed me into this, his original work. It has been a pleasure to work with him, and an apprenticeship in wisdom as well. Thanks to Madison Trammel and Pam Pugh for your encouragement and patience with me. Drs. Michael DeRoche, Gloria Halverson, Jeffrey Keenan, and Louis T. Riley, and embryologist Carol Sommerfelt added much to my understanding. (Any errors in the text are mine.) I thank C. Ben Mitchell for his constancy as an able advisor and friend. The Board of Directors of the Tennessee Center for Bioethics and Culture has been gracious regarding my taking time away to work on this project: Thank you. Lindy Fowler and Cile Cowan, dear friends, have provided well-timed support and encouragement. Finally, I thank my family for your love, support, and patience as I have worked on this project. To my husband, Louis, sons Ian, Tristan, and Grant, and daughter-in-law, Michaela: my heartfelt gratitude for your lives as well as your gifts to me.